NELSON'S

CORE
ADVANTAGE

TOM DANIELSON'S
CORE ADVANTAGE

CORE STRENGTH FOR CYCLING'S WINNING EDGE

Tom Danielson & Allison Westfahl

VELO press

BOULDER,
COLORADO

▼velopress®

3002 Sterling Circle, Suite 100
Boulder, Colorado 80301-2338 USA
(303) 440-0601 · Fax (303) 444-6788 · E-mail velopress@competitorgroup.com

Distributed in the United States and Canada by Ingram Publisher Services

Library of Congress Cataloging-in-Publication Data
Danielson, Tom, 1978–
Tom Danielson's core advantage: strength routines for cycling's winning edge /
Tom Danielson and Allison Westfahl.—1st ed.
        p. cm.
Includes index.
ISBN 978-1-934030-97-4 (pbk.: alk. paper)
1. Cycling—Training. 2. Muscle strength. I. Westfahl, Allison. II. Title.
III. Title: Core advantage.
GV1048.D36 2013
796.6—dc23
                                2012042139

For information on purchasing VeloPress books,
please call (800) 811-4210, ext. 2138, or visit www.velopress.com.

This paper meets the requirements of ANSI/NISO Z39.48-1992 (Permanence of Paper).

Cover design by Rick Landers
Front cover photograph by Gilbert Dupuy; back cover photograph by Mark Johnson
Interior photographs by Brad Kaminski except author photographs by Casey B. Gibson (p. 205)
    and Kirsten Boyer (p. 206)
Illustrations by Charlie Layton
Interior design and composition by Vicki Hopewell

Text set in Sentinel

13 14 15 / 10 9 8 7 6 5 4 3 2 1

CONTENTS

FOREWORD

Cycling has always represented freedom to me. The bike has been a tangible grounding mechanism that has stayed with me from an early age through major life changes and has come to be a foundational element of who I am. My relationship with cycling started when I was 12, growing up in Maine; I would ride around for hours, exploring the roads and indulging my curiosity for finding out "what's out there." As I matured and changed, my relationship with cycling also evolved. Today, cycling represents not only a tool for maintaining my fitness and pushing my physical boundaries but also a way for me to unplug from the demands of a frantic Hollywood lifestyle.

One of the ways that my enthusiasm for cycling has been expressed is through my love of professional cycling. It was in this arena that I first met Tommy D. I have always been a big fan and supporter of the Tour of California, and I had the pleasure of meeting Tom at the 2010 race. Our first conversation was brief, but even from that initial interaction I could tell that Tom shared my deep infatuation with the bike. It was clear that Tom's relationship with the sport of cycling was much more than simply a professional obligation.

It was this connection that led me to ask Tom to make an appearance in the 2011 Dempsey Challenge. The annual Dempsey Challenge is an international fund-raising platform in Lewiston/Auburn, Maine, which benefits The Patrick Dempsey Center for Cancer Hope & Healing at Central Maine Medical Center. At the 2011 event, Tom and I had a chance to spend more time together, and I told him to please call me if he ever found himself in Southern California in need of a training partner. Much to my delight, my phone rang just a few weeks later. That was the first of countless training rides that Tom and I would go on over the next year.

Given Tom's stature in the world of professional cycling, I was not surprised to witness just how strong he is on the bike. As an actor, I'm expected to stay in shape for the camera, so I'm no stranger to tough workouts and long hours in the gym. However, trying to keep up with Tom took my workouts to a whole new level! We both like to have fun while riding, but we're also both willing to work hard to get better, and Tom's level of excellence really inspired me to challenge my own limits on the bike. Tom shared with me that one of his secret weapons is core strength, and that his trainer Allison had designed some unique workouts that were specifically geared toward cycling. He showed me some of the exercises, and I immediately adopted them into my own routine.

When Tom told me that he was writing a book that contained all these core exercises, I knew it would be no ordinary workout book. Tom likes preparing for his sport as much as he likes participating in it—the training, the research, and the implementation are all part of his commitment to cycling. This book is a perfect reflection of Tom's detailed, well-studied approach to training.

The simple fact that you are reading this foreword indicates two things: You're a cyclist, and you're serious about progressing in the sport. By adopting the innovative ideas found in this work, I have little doubt that your skills on the bike will see drastic improvements—improvements that will be obvious to your friends as you leave them behind on your favorite ride!

—Patrick Dempsey

PREFACE

As a professional cyclist, I have always known how important it is to spend my daylight hours training on the bike. No matter what, time on the bike comes first. Raining? Go ride my bike. Sick? Go ride my bike. Burned out, sore, and unmotivated? Go ride my bike. Injured? Well . . . sit on my couch and wish I could go ride my bike.

In the fall of 2007 I was in a horrible bike crash during the Vuelta a España. I shattered my glenoid cavity—a part of the shoulder joint—and herniated the L5-S1 disc in my back. I had just signed a new contract with Slipstream Sports, which is based in Boulder, Colorado, and shortly after the crash I moved to Boulder from my former base in Durango, Colorado, in quite a broken state. Not only was I getting used to a new town and a new team, but I also didn't have my coaches and therapists whom I had grown to know and trust back in Durango. I needed some major rehab on my back and shoulder, so I started doing everything possible to get better—physical therapy, dry needling, massage, chiropractic. But nothing was working, and my injuries were becoming a huge liability. I needed to get healed and get back on the bike.

I heard through word of mouth that there was a trainer in Boulder named Allison Westfahl who had a real knack for fixing injuries in endurance athletes. I met with Allison in February 2008 and was immediately impressed with how she looked at the big picture instead of just focusing on the site of the injury. With her extensive background in physiology and her understanding of how the human body works during sports, she was able to diagnose muscular weaknesses and imbalances that were at the root of my injury.

Allison wanted to know my lifelong history of injuries, and I realized that my low back had actually been a problem for a long time. She had me do a little series of movements while she walked around me with a clipboard taking notes. After about 30 seconds, she said, "Okay, I know what's wrong. Your glute max isn't firing correctly, and your psoas is tight and overworked. Plus you have thoracic kyphosis, and your shoulder will never heal correctly if we don't fix that."

I reminded her that the pain was in my low back, not my glutes, but she insisted that fixing the source of the injury instead of just the site of the pain was the best approach. She said I should strengthen my core muscles in order to solve my injuries. Great, I thought. More crunches and back extensions. I had been put on "core strengthening" programs for years, and none had ever seemed to make a difference. But I decided to give it a chance since I was already there.

What happened in that first training session was a core workout like I'd never experienced. Allison had me do exercises that involved balance, coordination, and muscular endurance, all in positions that are similar to being on the bike. I did core exercises that I had never seen before, and I left feeling as if I had actually done a workout that made sense for cycling. The pain from my herniated disc started going away within two weeks, and after just four weeks of following Allison's core strengthening protocol I was completely pain-free.

Although I had gone to Allison just to recover from injury, we soon started talking about how following a core strengthening program year-round could really help me increase my power and performance on the bike. I was skeptical at first because lots of people had given me all kinds of advice over the years that never yielded any concrete results. "Do this, and you'll increase your power and performance on the bike." "Drink this tea; it will help your performance." "Sleep in this altitude tent, eat this food, ride this bike . . . blah, blah, blah." Everyone always had the magic answer, but it all seemed like a gimmick to me. However, I decided to give Allison a shot, because her program had indeed helped me recover from my injury, and in the process I realized that I was also stronger on my bike. I began to think that maybe if she could fix other areas of weakness in my riding the same way she had fixed my injury, then we would really be on to something.

That was at the beginning of 2008, and I have been working with Allison ever since. Communication has always been key for us. I told her I wanted to work on creating acceleration as I transition from in the saddle to out, and I wanted to be able to maintain power out of the saddle for long stretches. She would watch me ride so that she could identify which muscle groups weren't working at their optimum during certain points in my pedal stroke, and then she would come up with original exercises to fix the problem. Because a lot of the exercises were new, we had some fun naming them according to which ride or race had inspired them. We hope you'll get a kick out of the names as well!

By the beginning of 2012, Allison and I had amassed quite a storehouse of really effective, original core exercises. We decided that we wanted to share the exercises and programs with cyclists around the world, so that everyone could experience riding powerfully and pain-free.

The 50 exercises and 15 programs that you'll find in this book are the real deal. I've suffered through all of them and continue to do so. My hope is that you will use this book to become a better cyclist and to gain a deeper understanding of how a strong core can truly give you a winning edge.

—Tom Danielson

ACKNOWLEDGMENTS

Over the years of pursuing my dream in professional cycling, I have always loved sharing the things I have learned along the way. With the successes and failures has come a wealth of knowledge. I can't thank Allison enough for giving me the vision for us to write this book together. I love helping others become better cyclists, and Allison has enabled me to do it on a very large scale with this book.

I would like to share my appreciation of the team at VeloPress for being a company full of true athletes and cyclists. Because of this they were able to see the value in this project and not push it to the side, thinking it was just another way for a pro athlete to make some money. One more shout-out goes to my editor, Ted Costantino, for being lenient about my professional racing and training schedule. In a business full of timeliness and deadlines, Ted stayed calm and confident that I would get my tasks done no matter where in the world I was.

My family has also been very supportive and encouraging throughout. After my six-hour days on the bike, they had to endure my not being present while I worked on this book. I had no idea how much goes into writing a book like this, and I thank my wife, Stephanie, and my children for being patient with me as I learned the process.

—*Tom Danielson*

When Tom and I first starting talking about doing a project together, I never dreamed that the end result would be a book published by VeloPress. My sincerest thanks and gratitude to the team at Velo for giving us this opportunity and for letting us have complete creative control the entire way. Special thanks to Ted Costantino for enduring my attempts at physiology humor and to Charlie Layton and Brad Kaminski for translating the images in my head onto paper.

My friends, family, colleagues, and clients have all been incredibly supportive and encouraging during this process, especially my husband, Brian. Thank you for not complaining when I brought my laptop in the car, on vacation, to birthday parties, to the dog park, etc.

A special acknowledgment goes to Tom. It takes a unique combination of trust, respect, and mutual deference to allow an endurance athlete and a strength training coach to get along. Working with Tom has given me the chance to use my creativity to generate original exercises and programs, which has in turn made me a better trainer. Thanks, Tommy D.

—*Allison Westfahl*

WHAT IS
CORE
STRENGTH?

PART I

Core Strength Means Better Results

"Core strength." Once practically unheard-of, this term is now so widely used in the world of sports and fitness that it has become easy to dismiss. Athletes, fitness experts, and weekend warriors talk incessantly about how they are working on building their core, learning how to use core strength, and "just learned the most killer core routine, dude—you've gotta try it!" Health clubs offer core strength classes, fitness videos promise stronger core muscles, and we all probably agree that better core strength would probably—definitely—improve our fitness, solve our problems at work, and make us better people.

The truth is, core strength may not instantly make you a better citizen, but it will definitely make you a better cyclist. A regular regimen of core strength exercises will train your muscles and joints to work at their highest efficiency when you are cycling, and it will reduce your chances of injury. A strong core will stabilize your muscle paths to improve your transmission of power from your hips and legs to the pedals of your bike. Core strength will also improve your acceleration, and not only in a sprint; it will also make a significant difference in the hundreds of big and small accelerations that occur constantly in a fast-moving pace line or group. Additionally, solid core strength will improve your climbing and descending skills.

Before we show you how core strength can make you a better cyclist, though, there are some simpler points surrounding core strength that we should address, such as what exactly is the core? And what makes the core so special that you need a bunch of specific exercises—not to mention a whole book—to take care of it?

Understanding the Term "Core"

The term "core strength," while widely used, still causes a lot of confusion; many people mistakenly believe that "abdominals" and "core" are interchangeable terms. The abdominals consist of four muscles, all of which are located primarily on the anterior, or front, side of the body (Figure 1.1). The one exception is the transversus abdominis, which wraps around to the back side of the body.

The core consists of these abdominals *plus* all the other muscles that attach to the spine and the pelvis. In terms of geography, the core starts at the top of the torso and runs all the way to the bottom of the pelvis. That's a large area, and it houses countless muscle groups (Figure 1.2).

Included in these groups are muscles you may have previously categorized as being "lower-body" or "upper-body" muscles, such as the gluteals and latissimus dorsi. While these muscles are indeed part of the lower and upper body, respectively, they serve a dual function as part of the core, because they have either an origin or an insertion into the spine or pelvis. The terms "origin" and "insertion" refer to the parts of the body that anchor the muscle on each end. The origin is typically the proximal point (closest to the spine), and it tends to cover a large area, while the insertion is the distal point (farthest from the spine) and tends to cover a small area. When a muscle contracts, the origin and insertion move closer together, and when a muscle stretches, they move apart.

For example, the gluteus maximus (glute max) has an origin along the entire posterior gluteal line, which includes parts of the sacrum, ilium, coccyx, and sacrotuberous ligament. The muscle then fans out and inserts into the iliotibial tract and the gluteal tuberosity (Figure 1.3). When the glute max is contracted, the origin and insertion move closer together, causing the hip to extend and externally rotate. The

FIGURE 1.1 **ABDOMINAL MUSCLES**

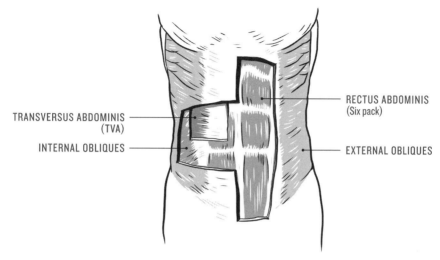

TRANSVERSUS ABDOMINIS (TVA)

INTERNAL OBLIQUES

RECTUS ABDOMINIS (Six pack)

EXTERNAL OBLIQUES

reason this movement is considered to be a "core movement" is because the pelvis is involved; the glute max must help stabilize the pelvis while the hip is being extended.

The actual number of muscles that originate and/or insert into the spine and pelvis is still up for debate, mainly because no one can agree on whether to count groups of muscles as one muscle or to name each one individually. For example, the hamstrings (which originate in the pelvis and are therefore part of the core) consist of three different muscles, but are almost always referred to as a singular "hamstring." There is also the nagging question of whether large areas of fascia found in the core should be counted as core "muscles." Regardless of these debates, the muscles belonging to the core are vastly greater in both number and scope than those included in the category of "abs."

It is often thought that the sole purpose of core muscles is to keep the middle part of the body stable, but this is only a small part of their mission; Table 1.1 lists the various functions of the muscles that make up the core. Core muscles also generate power to the arms and legs, they protect the spine and pelvis from injury, and they help maintain good posture. Keeping the core muscles in tip-top shape is a good idea for everyone in general, but even more so for cyclists. Because cycling is performed in a semi-prone (facedown) position with the trunk of the body all squished up, the

FIGURE 1.2 **CORE MUSCLES**

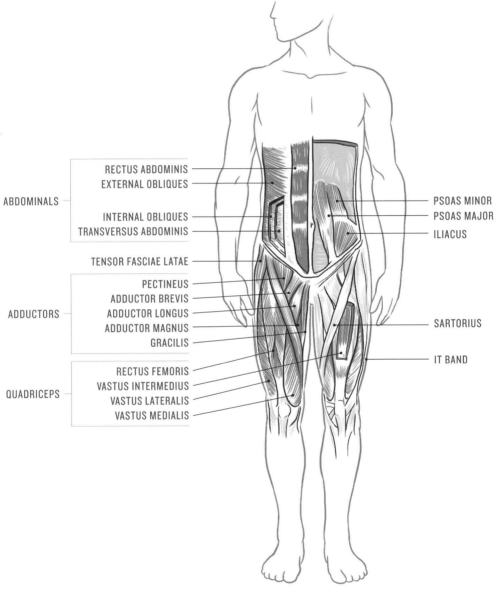

ABDOMINALS
RECTUS ABDOMINIS
EXTERNAL OBLIQUES
INTERNAL OBLIQUES
TRANSVERSUS ABDOMINIS
TENSOR FASCIAE LATAE

ADDUCTORS
PECTINEUS
ADDUCTOR BREVIS
ADDUCTOR LONGUS
ADDUCTOR MAGNUS
GRACILIS

QUADRICEPS
RECTUS FEMORIS
VASTUS INTERMEDIUS
VASTUS LATERALIS
VASTUS MEDIALIS

PSOAS MINOR
PSOAS MAJOR
ILIACUS

SARTORIUS

IT BAND

ANTERIOR

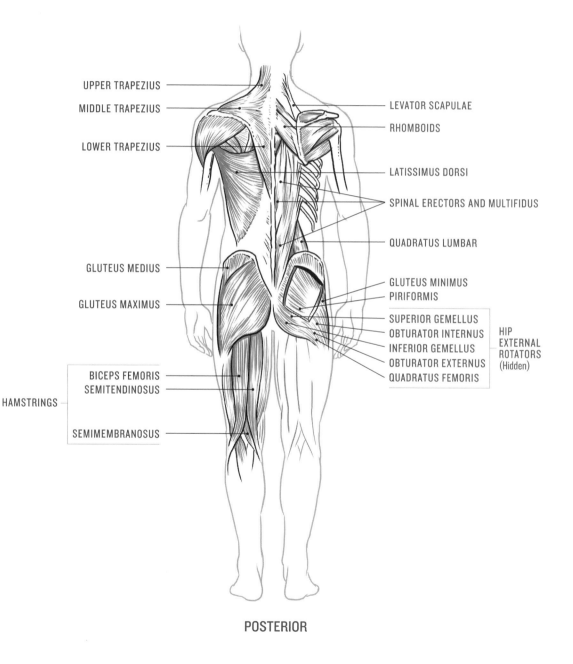

UPPER TRAPEZIUS

MIDDLE TRAPEZIUS

LOWER TRAPEZIUS

LEVATOR SCAPULAE

RHOMBOIDS

LATISSIMUS DORSI

SPINAL ERECTORS AND MULTIFIDUS

QUADRATUS LUMBAR

GLUTEUS MEDIUS

GLUTEUS MAXIMUS

GLUTEUS MINIMUS

PIRIFORMIS

SUPERIOR GEMELLUS

OBTURATOR INTERNUS

INFERIOR GEMELLUS

OBTURATOR EXTERNUS

QUADRATUS FEMORIS

HIP EXTERNAL ROTATORS (Hidden)

BICEPS FEMORIS

SEMITENDINOSUS

HAMSTRINGS

SEMIMEMBRANOSUS

POSTERIOR

TOMMY'S TAKE Redemption time. That's what Stage 3 of the 2012 USA Pro Challenge was for me. I was just coming off a terrible crash less than two months earlier in the Tour de France (see Chapter 2 for the full story), and I think a lot of people may have questioned whether I would be ready for the Pro Challenge. But Colorado is the state where I live and train, and I know the routes well, because I've ridden them many times, so I thought that if I could just come into the race with some solid strength and conditioning, I might actually have a chance. Turns out I got that chance during stage 3 from Gunnison to Aspen.

Our team strategy for that day was aggressive but simple: Get two guys in the first breakaway and create a 3- to 4-minute gap right from the start. Then I would attack out of the peloton and hopefully go across to the breakaway on the first climb. My teammates Dave Zabriskie and Nathan Haas were in that first breakaway. When I attacked over the top of the first climb I was going a bit faster than the rest of the 22 guys in the breakaway, so Zabriskie and Haas had to lift the pace a bit in order to maintain the 4-minute gap over the peloton. Dave stayed with me for the next 70 miles until the last climb. At the bottom of Independence Pass, I pulled ahead and essentially did the last 80 km of the race by myself.

Going it alone in front of my fans in my home state was an experience I will never forget. I didn't know if I was capable of holding it the whole time; among other things, there was a lot of wind. I just took it moment by moment and set little goals for myself. Independence Pass is an icon of Colorado, and to be solo for such a long way was a special experience for me.

That day I really stressed my body, and at every moment I was expecting the next second to be the one where I lost my strength or pedal rhythm. But I was amazed at how all the hard work I had done on my core allowed me to keep my composure. It's one thing to win in a solo breakaway and then be crushed for the rest of the race, but I had my best cycling performance ever in my home state, and I even went on to win the title of Most Aggressive Rider.

demands on the core musculature are magnified, and so are the consequences of letting your core muscles become weak (Figure 1.4).

Any weakness in the core can inhibit your performance on the bike. Unfortunately, most cyclists suffer from several problems related to muscle weakness, because they tend to feed off each other. Muscular imbalances can lead to overuse injuries and poor posture; overuse injuries can cause decreased power production

FIGURE 1.3 **ORIGIN AND INSERTION OF THE GLUTEUS MAXIMUS**

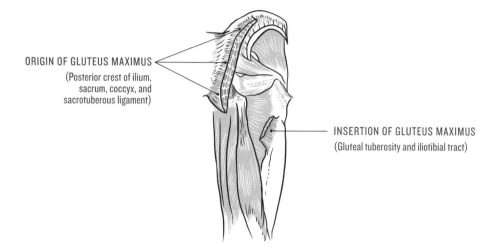

ORIGIN OF GLUTEUS MAXIMUS
(Posterior crest of ilium,
sacrum, coccyx, and
sacrotuberous ligament)

INSERTION OF GLUTEUS MAXIMUS
(Gluteal tuberosity and iliotibial tract)

in the legs; poor posture can cause muscular imbalances. It quickly becomes difficult to identify which problem occurred first, which one is the worst, and how to go
about fixing things. The first step in combating performance-depleting problems is
to examine your current program to make sure you aren't accidentally exacerbating
the problem by doing inappropriate exercises.

Stop Doing Crunches!

Due to the misperception that only the abdominal muscles constitute the core, exercise
routines commonly focus on strengthening those four abdominals, sometimes to the
exclusion of all others. But each muscle of the true core has a specific function, making
it important to achieve optimum strength in all the muscles, not just the abdominals.

Multiple problems can arise when the abdominals are strengthened and the
remainder of the core is ignored; chief among these problems are muscular imbalances. When an imbalance occurs in the muscular system, a muscle or a group of
muscles becomes dominant and overactive, while a different muscle becomes weak
and inactive. The imbalance throws off the carefully designed system of duties for
which each muscle is responsible.

FIGURE 1.4 **CONSEQUENCES OF WEAK CORE MUSCLES**

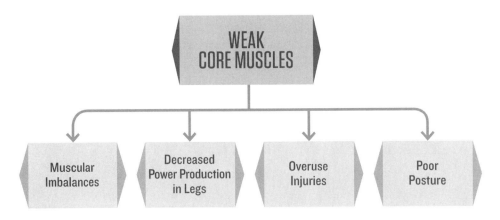

One of the most common imbalances seen in the core musculature is the overdevelopment of the rectus abdominis, which in turn causes the transversus abdominis, psoas, and low back to become weak and inactive. How does the rectus abdominis become so dominant? Too many crunches.

Consider a traditional ab routine: You start with some basic crunches, move on to some side crunches, and finish up with some reverse crunches. Sounds like a pretty complete set of exercises, right? The harsh truth for cyclists is that crunches actually do much more harm than good. If you fit the profile of the typical cyclist, you probably already have an overworked and tight rectus abdominis (the "six-pack" muscle used during crunches) due to the amount of time you spend in a crunch position while riding. A steady diet of ab crunches only makes the problem worse.

The primary function of the rectus abdominis is to shorten the length between the rib cage and the pelvis, which is an effective way to achieve an aerodynamic position on the bike. Off the bike, however, shortening the rectus abdominis over and over—which is what happens during a crunch—will encourage poor posture and put excessive pressure on the discs of the lumbar spine. Think about it: If you perform a crunch while standing up, you have to hunch your shoulders forward and stoop over in order to flex your abs.

Another problem with traditional crunches is that they are performed while lying on your back, thereby training your abdominal muscles to fire when the rest of your body is being stabilized by the floor. How many times do you actually use your abdominal muscles this way in real life? Probably never. Would you ever train for a ride by lying on your back and pedaling your legs up in the air? Of course not, because this type of training would never directly translate into improved performance on the bike.

As previously mentioned, the larger problem with a crunch-based routine is that it creates muscular imbalances, which in turn decrease the body's ability to generate optimum stability and power on the bike. When a muscle (in this case, the rectus abdominis) is overdeveloped, it effectively starts bullying the muscles around it, making those muscles incapable of doing their jobs. The muscles of the core that are most commonly bullied into submission are the transversus abdominis, the internal obliques, and the muscles of the low back. These muscles are the primary providers of stabilization to the pelvis and spine during movement; when they aren't functioning at full capacity, their ability to help the body move with optimum power and efficiency is drastically decreased.

In order for the muscles of the core to do their job, each muscle must be equally strong—no bullies allowed. The only way to accomplish this muscular balance is to take crunches off the field so that the other players get a chance to see some game time.

The notion of doing a core strength routine without crunches may seem blasphemous. As a vanity-obsessed nation, we have all been brainwashed from childhood to believe that crunches are good for us and that an Adonis-like six-pack is the ultimate sign of strength. Heck, even the president's physical fitness test for schoolchildren includes a section that counts the number of curl-ups (another name for a crunch) that can be done in one minute! But now it's time to set aside that old approach, step away from the ab crunch machine, and start working on the entire core.

TOMMY'S TAKE All the core work I did before meeting Allison was based on doing crunches. I got pretty good at doing crunches, but they didn't ever make me feel like a stronger cyclist. In fact, they made me more hunched over and contributed to my low-back pain.

TABLE 1.1 FUNCTIONS OF THE CORE MUSCLES

MUSCLE	CORE FUNCTION
HAMSTRINGS *Consist of the biceps femoris, semimembranosus, and semitendinosus.*	Extends hips; stabilizes low back and pelvis during movement.
QUADRICEPS *Consists of the rectus femoris, vastus lateralis, vastus medius, and vastus intermedius. Rectus femoris is also categorized as a "hip-flexor muscle."*	Flexes hips; stabilizes pelvis during movement.
HIP ADDUCTOR COMPLEX *Consists of the adductor magnus, adductor longus, adductor brevis, pectineus, and gracilis.*	Flexes and internally rotates the femur; assists with hip extension.
HIP ABDUCTOR COMPLEX *Consists of the gluteus medius, gluteus minimus, and tensor fasciae latae (TFL). The TFL is also categorized as a "hip-flexor muscle."*	Abducts (movement away from the body) the femur.
HIP EXTERNAL ROTATORS *Consists of the piriformis, quadratus femoris, gemellus superior, gemellus inferior, obturator internus, and obturator externus.*	Externally rotates and extends hips; stabilizes the pelvis and femur.
GLUTEUS MAXIMUS	Extends and externally rotates hips; stabilizes the SI joint.
ILIOPSOAS COMPLEX *Consists of the iliacus, psoas major, and psoas minor. Also categorized as a "hip-flexor muscle."*	Flexes hips; stabilizes the lumbar spine.
SPINAL ERECTORS AND MULTIFIDUS	Extends and stabilizes the spine.
LATISSIMUS DORSI	Stabilizes the thoracic and lumbar spine; stabilizes the pelvis.

MUSCLE	CORE FUNCTION
RHOMBOIDS	Retracts (pulling together) and downwardly rotates the shoulder blades.
TRAPEZIUS *Consists of the upper, middle, and lower trapezius.*	Extends and contralaterally rotates the cervical spine; retracts and depresses shoulder blades.
RECTUS ABDOMINIS *Also called the "six-pack."*	Flexes the spine; stabilizes the lumbar and pelvis.
TRANSVERSUS ABDOMINIS *Also known as the TVA.*	Produces intra-abdominal pressure; stabilizes the lumbar and pelvis during movement.
ABDOMINAL OBLIQUES *Consists of the internal and external obliques.*	Flexes and rotates the spine and pelvis; stabilizes the lumbar and pelvis.

Core Strength That Works for Cyclists

If you as a cyclist aren't supposed to be doing crunches, then what are you supposed to do? It's not enough to just randomly work all the muscles of the core and hope that useful core strength emerges. Instead, you need to work your core muscles in a functional manner so that their strength can be directly translated to the activity and demands of cycling.

So what is a "functional" core strength routine? Broadly, it is one that meets the criteria set out by the National Academy of Sports Medicine: "All functional movement patterns involve deceleration, stabilization, and acceleration, which occur at every joint in the kinetic chain and in all three planes of motion."

Perfectly clear, right? Okay, let's break it down. First of all, the overall thesis of functional training is that movements performed during training sessions should mimic movements performed in the sport for which you are training. For cycling, therefore, we need to train the muscles, joints, and soft tissue of your body to operate at their highest efficiency while you are riding. Put another way, the exercises in your core routine should focus on *specific movements* as opposed to *specific muscles*.

When you approach your core strength program in this way, it soon becomes obvious that lying on your back doing crunches is not really functional at all. Those crunches aren't going to get you anywhere near where you need to be in terms of balanced muscle strength and stability.

Instead, you need exercises that qualify as functional. To get there, let's look at the terms that help define functional training.

Deceleration

Deceleration (also known as the eccentric muscle contraction) refers to the body's ability to safely and effectively slow down a movement. As its name implies, deceleration puts the brakes on whatever action is being performed. Don't worry, this kind of deceleration won't slow down your cycling. It will, however, slow down your rate of injury. If a muscle can't safely and efficiently slow down after it is put into motion, it will eventually move past its limit and tear. Think about the implications of driving a car with no brake pedal: The acceleration would continue on forever, and eventually the car would crash into something and sustain damage. The same is true of human movement.

The ramifications of poor or improper deceleration in musculature can best be exemplified by the number of anterior cruciate ligament, or ACL, tears that are sustained. Although the ACL is not part of the core, the hamstrings, the muscle group often responsible for ACL injuries, is an integral part of your core architecture. Of the approximately 200,000 ACL tears that occur each year, 80 percent are noncontact, meaning that the injury was sustained without contact or impact from another person or object. A noncontact ACL tear can almost always be attributed to poor hamstring strength. The hamstrings are responsible for decelerating knee extension during pivoting or landing from a jumping motion. This is a prime example of how weakness in a core muscle can potentially lead to injury.

TOMMY'S TAKE The idea of learning to squat properly seemed ridiculous to me until I understood how it could affect my power when I'm getting in and out of the saddle. It has always been easy for me to generate power when I'm going from in the saddle to out of the saddle, but when I go from out to back in, I tend to have a 2- to 3-second lull in my power output. Once my body readjusts to the seated position, I regain my power. By improving my core strength—specifically my ability to use my core to decelerate my body properly when I'm transitioning back into the saddle—I have been able to get rid of that lull and essentially keep the gas on the entire time. If you don't lose power every time you transition back into the saddle, you will gain a real edge over your competition.

Given that cycling doesn't require quick pivoting or jumping motions, you may be thinking you're off the hook in terms of needing your hamstring muscles to provide deceleration. After all, almost every person you know who has torn an ACL did it while playing soccer, basketball, or skiing. While you may not be in danger of sustaining a knee injury from running around a field kicking a ball, you probably perform a basic squat countless times throughout the day, and this movement requires deceleration from the hamstrings in order to slow down the rate at which the knee extends when you rise and the rate at which the hip flexes forward when you squat (Figure 1.5). Without proper deceleration, your body could move upward too quickly, putting the joints of the hips and knees in danger.

Still not convinced you need to know how to squat as a cyclist? Do you ever stand up out of the saddle while riding and then sit back down? If the answer is yes, then you need to know how to squat properly.

Stabilization

The second aspect of a functional exercise is stabilization, otherwise known as isometric muscular contraction. A muscle is working isometrically when it is held at a fixed length instead of actively lengthening or shortening. By holding a muscle at a fixed length, the joints at either end are stabilized.

FIGURE 1.5 **CORE MUSCLES USED DURING A SQUAT**

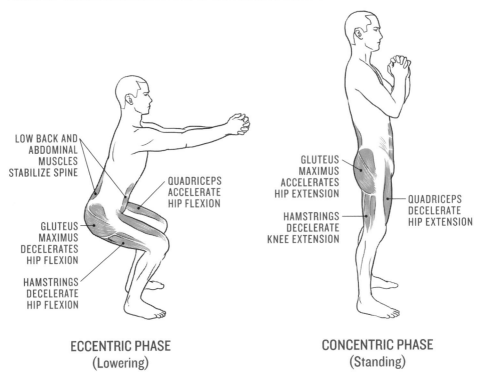

LOW BACK AND ABDOMINAL MUSCLES STABILIZE SPINE

QUADRICEPS ACCELERATE HIP FLEXION

GLUTEUS MAXIMUS DECELERATES HIP FLEXION

HAMSTRINGS DECELERATE HIP FLEXION

GLUTEUS MAXIMUS ACCELERATES HIP EXTENSION

QUADRICEPS DECELERATE HIP EXTENSION

HAMSTRINGS DECELERATE KNEE EXTENSION

ECCENTRIC PHASE
(Lowering)

CONCENTRIC PHASE
(Standing)

In a traditional approach to strength training, stabilization is often supplied by a machine, a bench, or some other stable surface that supports the body. With functional training, stabilization is provided by the body itself, and it is provided both isometrically (body not moving) and dynamically (body in motion). It may seem odd to think of core muscles providing stabilization while the body is in motion, but this is exactly the capacity in which they must function when you're on the bike. Each time you push down on a pedal, your core muscles have to provide dynamic stabilization so that your body remains stable while the bike is moving forward underneath it. Without proper stabilization, your spine and pelvis would be moving all over the place while you ride, which would not only put you in danger of falling off your bike, but would also decrease your ability to effectively transmit power from the core muscles out to the extremities.

Acceleration

Finally, there's the aspect of functional strength training that interests all cyclists: acceleration. When you want to go faster on your bike, you increase the pace at which you are pedaling. This action happens in a split second, but it is the result of a very complex chain of neuromuscular events, one of which is a concentric muscle contraction, otherwise known as acceleration. Contrary to an eccentric contraction (or deceleration), a concentric muscle contraction shortens the muscle fiber. Earlier we looked at how the hamstring muscles work eccentrically to decelerate the rate at which you stand up from a squat position. Now let's look at what the hamstring muscles do when they are shortening, or accelerating.

When the hamstring muscles contract and shorten, their main job is to assist with hip extension and knee flexion. Hip extension happens every time you take a step and push off the ground with your foot, every time you stand up from a seated position, and every time you push your foot behind your body. In cycling, hip extension

TOMMY'STAKE I had a tough lesson in muscle contraction velocity at the 2012 Vuelta País Vasco in Spain. As I started preparing for the 2012 season, I spent so much time on my regular road bike trying to increase my power that I ended up neglecting my time trial (TT) bike. When I showed up at the Vuelta País Vasco, my fitness on my road bike was pretty exceptional, so I assumed my fitness on my TT bike would be the same, even though I hadn't devoted much time to it. To my surprise, when I got into my time trial, my power meter was reading really low, and I had one of my worst time trials. I was pushing as hard as I could, but the power wasn't there—not even close. I believe the reason for that is the muscles that enable me to produce power in a time trial position weren't firing correctly because they weren't used to being fired in that extended position.

In time trialing, because of the position that you're in, it is really important to be able to access the full muscle contraction velocity when you're in a hyperextended position. So when I got back home to Boulder, Colorado, and started to train for the Tour of California, I focused on getting my hamstrings and glutes firing again on my TT bike, and the results paid off. I was on the podium largely because I had my full muscle contraction velocity available during every stage of the race.

happens as you extend your foot downward, and knee flexion happens when you pull your foot back up. This is why hamstrings are the main muscles working during your upstroke, and why your hamstrings always seem to scream when you start focusing on pulling up on the pedals instead of pushing down.

An important tenet of concentric muscle contractions is that the contraction velocity (acceleration) is inversely proportional to the load placed on the muscle. What this means in bike speak is that the lighter the load you place on a muscle, the faster it can contract. You can test this yourself: Start riding on a flat straightaway in a very low gear (little to no resistance), then gradually start to shift into higher gears (adding resistance) but try to maintain the same cadence. Eventually you won't be able to keep the cadence you started with because your muscles cannot contract at the same speed; the load placed on the muscles has increased, and, consequently, the speed at which they can fire has decreased. One of the many talents that distinguish world-class cyclists is that they have the ability to maintain a very high pedaling cadence, even when the muscle is under a high load or force.

Core Strength in All Planes of Motion

Understanding how the terms "deceleration," "stabilization," and "acceleration" can affect your core training is definitely useful, but what truly differentiates functional core strength training from traditional core strength training is that all three of these movement variables happen in multiple planes of motion (Figure 1.6).

With a traditional approach to strength training, muscles are frequently isolated and worked in a stable, controlled environment through one plane of motion. Take the standard bench press as an example; during this exercise, the athlete lies on his or her back on a bench and pushes a bar loaded with weights toward the ceiling. While this exercise has the potential to build muscle mass and increase the force production of the chest and shoulder muscles (pectorals and deltoids), the benefits pretty much stop there. In other words, an exercise like the bench press may give you nice-looking muscles for the beach, but it won't necessarily improve your ability to use those muscles to efficiently perform daily movements, activities, and sports.

FIGURE 1.6 **PLANES OF MOTION**

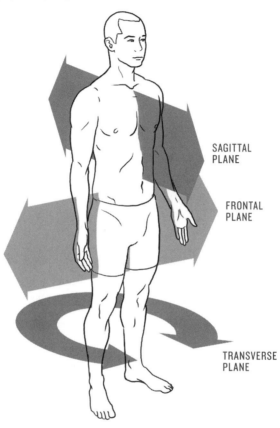

SAGITTAL
PLANE

FRONTAL
PLANE

TRANSVERSE
PLANE

What many traditional exercises ultimately fail to deliver is a solid connection between the nervous and muscular systems. Sticking with the example of the bench press, let's take a look at the number of joints and muscles involved and the plane of motion in which they are used. The primary muscle used (agonist) is the pectoralis major, with additional strength (synergists) being provided by the anterior deltoid, pectoralis minor, and biceps brachii. Absent from this scene are stabilizing and neutralizing muscles; the body is already stabilized and neutralized by the bench, which means the muscles that would ordinarily do this work are allowed to shut off or underperform during the movement.

Furthermore, the bar used in a traditional bench press is straight, meaning that the path the arms must follow to complete the movement is already determined by the straightness of the bar. When a movement is performed in a predicted, stable pattern, it only has to move through a single plane of motion, in this case, the sagittal plane.

This type of training would be very useful if we used our pectoral muscles in a single plane of motion during daily movements, but we don't. In fact, we rarely use any muscle in a single, predicted plane of motion. And therein lies the entire foundation of functional training: To strengthen core muscles, exercises must mimic the actual movement in which you will use those muscles to perform activities or sports. By choosing core exercises that are functional and specific to the sport of cycling, you will avoid wasting time on exercises that don't improve your performance.

How can you tell the difference between a functional core exercise and a traditional core exercise? Functional exercises will require the body to provide its own stabilization (no benches or machines), will work in multiple planes of motion, and will ask the muscles to speed up (acceleration), hold still (stabilization), and slow down (deceleration). Table 1.2 lists some examples of how to tell the difference between traditional and functional core exercises. You can find descriptions and explanations of the functional exercises in Part II.

TABLE 1.2 COMPARISON OF TRADITIONAL VS. FUNCTIONAL CORE EXERCISES

TRADITIONAL	FUNCTIONAL
Hamstring curl machine	Hip Bridges *(see p. 109)*
Seated row machine	Shoulder Blade Squeeze *(see p. 110)*
Abdominal crunch	Mountain Climbers *(see p. 111)*
Adductor/abductor machine	Crossover Squats *(see p. 140)*

Using Core Strength for Balance on the Bike

One of the most important performance benefits you can receive from functional core strength is improved balance. By increasing the functional strength of your core, you are also improving your neuromuscular efficiency, one of the key players in achieving better balance.

Neuromuscular efficiency refers to the ability of the nervous system to properly recruit the correct muscles to control movement throughout all three planes of motion. By increasing the rate at which your nervous system can respond to outside forces such as gravity, ground reaction forces, momentum, and the movement of other muscles, you will also increase your balance. After all, balance is really just a reaction to something else that is going on.

For example, every time you take a step forward, your body must react to the force from the ground, the speed at which you are moving forward, and the power generated by muscles contracting. Without balance, you would fall over just walking.

For cyclists, balance stabilizes the body and the bike, and it must be achieved both isometrically (not moving) and dynamically (in motion). Isometric balance on the bike is needed in several scenarios: descending, stopping, or any other time you are holding your position steady atop the bike without moving your arms or legs. To achieve true isometric balance, each muscle in the core needs to contribute the proper amount of work. If there is a weak link in the chain, the weakness will be transmitted to the neighboring muscles, which can have devastating effects if you need to call upon your core to provide isometric stabilization when you're bombing downhill at 40 mph and hit a pothole.

Dynamic balance is just as crucial as isometric balance. Dynamic balance is often a difficult concept to understand, mainly because the traditional definition of "balance" involves holding something perfectly still and steady. A functional approach to core strength, however, recognizes that balance happens both while the body is held still and while it is in motion.

Even a basic movement like pedaling requires more dynamic stabilization than you may think. There are 29 muscles that connect to the lumbo-pelvic-hip complex, all of which are working together while pedaling to not only push the bike forward

TOMMY'S TAKE
Being able to stabilize your bike and your body when you're out of the saddle has more benefits than just keeping you upright. Most people would agree that when they get out of the saddle their heart rate jumps. In my case, however, I'm able to get out of the saddle without having it affect my heart rate too much because I'm able to stabilize my bike with my core.

When you're climbing out of the saddle, you want to be able to use both your upper and lower body to create a rhythmic bounce. If you don't have an efficient core, you won't be able to maintain that bounce for long periods of time, because your arms will be working to hold your body up, and your legs will be working the pedals, but they will be working independently. Having a strong core helps to establish a good neuromuscular relationship between the arms and legs, and that relationship will help keep your heart rate down, because you will waste less energy. The stronger the core, the longer you can stay out of the saddle without having your heart rate skyrocket.

but also to keep you from tipping over as you ride. If the muscles of the core can't hold your pelvis steady during a basic pedal stroke, your body will need to overcorrect to keep from tipping from side to side with each pedal stroke.

A more visual example of dynamic stabilization on the bike is climbing out of the saddle. With each pedal stroke executed out of the saddle, the muscles of the core must work to ensure the body stays stable atop the moving bike and that excess energy is not wasted moving from side to side. The deep core muscles are working to hold the spine and pelvis steady, allowing the muscles on the periphery of the core to move quickly and efficiently to push the pedals down over and over ... and over. If you have ever felt weak, unsteady, or just plain uncomfortable when climbing out of the saddle, a weak core may be the culprit. Once your core muscles are strengthened and firing correctly, you will be able to pop in and out of the saddle seamlessly without missing a pedal stroke.

Using Core Strength to Gain Power

It might seem difficult to believe that having strong, functional muscles in the center of your body could somehow increase the power output in your legs, but that's exactly what happens. By maintaining strong core musculature, you decrease your chances of experiencing what are commonly referred to as "energy leaks." An energy leak is a point where energy is lost during the transfer of force. Leaks occur most frequently in the torso and are the result of the body not being able to stabilize joints correctly. In other words, energy leaks are most often caused by weak core muscles that cannot properly stabilize the joints of the spine and pelvis.

A common energy leak in cyclists occurs at the lumbar spine, or low back. If the deep core muscles are not strong enough to stabilize the pelvis during a pedal stroke, the low back will flex and extend excessively each time you push your foot down. The result is that energy is "leaked" at the low back instead of being transferred to the glute max, which is a larger and stronger muscle capable of producing more force. As Mike Allen, the director of rehabilitation services at the Steadman Hawkins Clinic in Denver, notes, "Efficiency, power, and injury prevention are strongly dependent on the cyclist's ability to maintain proper alignment over extended periods of time. Low back and knee injuries commonly occur when alignment is compromised and energy is leaked to adjacent structures via compensation patterns. A well-developed trunk and hip strengthening program is essential for both performance and longevity."

A second important way in which the core provides power on the bike is by giving the legs a strong foundation from which to work. The large muscle groups of the legs (hamstrings, quadriceps, and gluteals) all originate at the pelvis; if the core muscles are weak, the pelvis will be unstable and the leg muscles will not be able to move with optimum efficiency. The core acts as a power conductor for the extremities, helping to maximize muscular efficiency and decrease wasted energy.

Finally, having strong extremity muscles (i.e., big quads and hamstrings) but a weak core will lead to inefficient movement patterns, causing a decrease in force production. When a muscle is so strong and dominant that it starts to take over the function of other muscles, it creates a scenario called "synergistic dominance." Every muscle in the body has a primary function, and when it's working in this capacity it is called the "agonist." For example, the gluteus maximus is the prime mover, or agonist, for hip extension. Hip extension happens for cyclists with every downward push on the pedals, so it's important that your body can perform this movement correctly.

> **TOMMY'S TAKE** Power is everything in cycling. Whoever can produce the most power for the longest period of time crosses the finish line first. To produce power and accelerate quickly, you have to pull up on one pedal with one leg at the same time you push down on the other, and it's imperative that no energy is lost in the core during this process. Cyclists talk all the time about how 1 percent power is the difference between first and tenth place; not losing energy through your core is that 1 percent.

While the glute max is working as the agonist, the hamstrings and the erector spinae (muscles that run along each side of the spine) are also working to assist in this movement, which makes them the synergists. It's very similar to how a baseball team works: Everyone has a position in which they specialize, and it's the job of each player to be the best he can be at that position while simultaneously working as a member of a team. But what would happen if the first baseman noticed that the pitcher was faltering a bit and he decided to take over that position? The pitcher would be wandering around the field without a job, first base would be left uncovered, the first baseman wouldn't be pitching very well (after all, it's not his specialty), and pretty soon the team would fall apart. Likewise, if the glute max (which is part of the core, remember) is not doing its job to extend the hip, the synergist muscles (hamstrings and erector spinae, in this case) will step in and dominate—hence the term "synergistic dominance." This is a problem not only because the hamstrings and erectors will eventually become injured from being overworked, but also because you will lose power and efficiency from not having the glute max on the job.

Get to Work!

The exercises and routines in this book focus on the core exercises that are most specific to cycling. All of the concepts discussed in this chapter have been assembled to create functional core strength training programs that will improve neuromuscular efficiency, strengthen muscles throughout multiple planes of motion, increase balance and coordination, and improve power production. If you want to be a better cyclist, it's time to start incorporating functional core strength training into your routine. It will take patience and diligence, and you will probably have some humbling moments (be sure to read Tommy's Takes on this subject in Part II), but your hard work will yield a strong, functional core that will help increase your performance on the bike.

CHAPTER 2

Common Injuries

If you know a cyclist who has never been injured, take a picture, because no one will believe you. Injuries are so prevalent among cyclists that it almost seems like fiction to hear about someone riding pain-free. Although cycling is a great way to get in shape without the side effects of high-impact sports like running, there is no getting around the fact that cyclists still suffer from an abnormally high rate of sport-induced pain.

The most commonly reported noncontact injuries are muscular overuse injuries and spinal disc injuries (Figure 2.1). Luckily, increasing your core strength can help lower your chances of incurring a noncontact injury and help you recover from injury if you're already suffering.

Muscular Overuse Injuries

Overuse injuries can be difficult to spot, because often the rider doesn't feel any pain until it's too late. A story frequently heard around the sports medicine clinic might sound something like this: "I don't know what happened—one day I was riding, and suddenly my outer knee started to hurt real bad. Now it hurts every time I ride."

FIGURE 2.1 **COMMON INJURIES FOUND IN CYCLISTS**

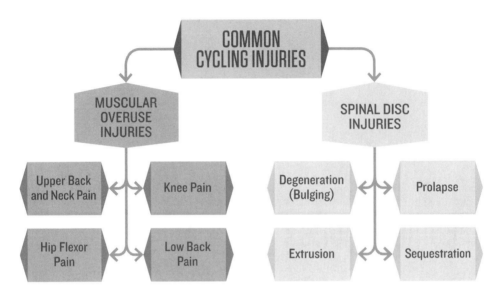

While it may seem like that pain came from out of the blue, it was probably building up over a period of time, slowly simmering until just the right amount of each ingredient was added and then—bam! A muscular overuse injury served up piping hot.

For cyclists, the parts of the body most prone to overuse injuries are the knees, hip flexors, low back, upper back, and neck. Sometimes an overuse injury is simply the result of too many hours in the saddle; muscles can only handle so much work before they get tired and shut down. But most of the time an overuse injury is the result of a muscle performing the wrong job, which excessively taxes the muscle and causes it to work too much—hence the term "overuse."

The process by which a muscle starts to perform the wrong job is complicated, but it almost always starts with a weak link in the core musculature. In this chapter you will learn which of the core muscles are most susceptible to weakness and how these weaknesses can lead to a self-perpetuating cycle of injury. Examining the process by which this happens will help provide a clear understanding of why keeping your core strong and healthy is essential for avoiding aches and pains on the bike.

HIP FLEXOR PAIN

If you find yourself sitting up during a ride and rubbing the area in front of your hip bones, you are the unwitting recipient of hip flexor overuse. When the hip flexor muscles are overused, they become inflamed, causing pain and cramping that can range from mildly uncomfortable to nearly debilitating. The pain typically becomes more pronounced when the hip flexors are excessively taxed, which happens as the upper body gets lower toward the knees (think time trial position) and when the amount of resistance placed on the hip flexors is increased (climbing and using a slow cadence).

As the injury matures, the pain will be noticeable every time hip flexion occurs, or every time the knees are raised toward the chest or the chest is lowered toward the knees. Because hip flexion happens with every pedal stroke, injuries can progress quickly. To avoid this nagging injury, we need to examine how hip flexor health can be increased with proper core conditioning.

Step one of understanding a hip flexor overuse injury is recognizing that the term "hip flexor" actually refers to a group of five muscles, all of which contribute to hip flexion. The fact that five muscles have to coordinate with each other is one of the reasons hip flexor injuries are so common; with that many players on the field, someone is bound to drop the ball. The five muscles that make up the hip flexors are the tensor fasciae latae, the rectus femoris (one of the four quadriceps muscles), the sartorius, the iliacus, and the psoas (Figure 2.2).

Cycling puts an extraordinary amount of strain on the hip flexors, because the upper body is leaning forward (hip flexion) while the knees are being brought up to the chest over and over again (also hip flexion). If you are riding with your hands in the drops or if you are bent over your time trial bars, your hip flexors will be shortened even more. When a muscle is subjected to chronic shortening, it will eventually lose its ability to extend back out to its full length unless a regular stretching routine is employed.

As a muscle loses its ability to extend and contract through its entire movement spectrum, the length-tension relationship of the muscle will be altered. Length-tension relationship refers to the length of a muscle fiber and the force it generates at that length (Figure 2.3). As a muscle becomes chronically shortened and tight, the

FIGURE 2.2 HIP FLEXOR MUSCLES WITH STRAIN ON PSOAS

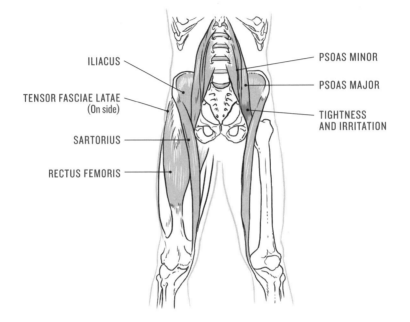

ILIACUS

TENSOR FASCIAE LATAE
(On side)

SARTORIUS

RECTUS FEMORIS

PSOAS MINOR

PSOAS MAJOR

TIGHTNESS
AND IRRITATION

FIGURE 2.3 OPTIMUM LENGTH-TENSION RELATIONSHIP OF A MUSCLE FIBER

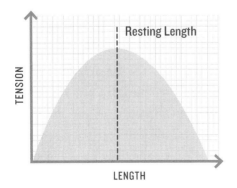

Resting Length

TENSION

LENGTH

FIGURE 2.4 SHORTENED LENGTH-TENSION RELATIONSHIP OF A MUSCLE FIBER

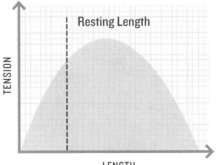

Resting Length

TENSION

LENGTH

line labeled "resting length" begins to move to the left, causing the tension, or force potential, of the muscle to decrease (Figure 2.4).

In the case of the hip flexors, the two that are prone to becoming the tightest during cycling are the psoas (pronounced "so-az") and iliacus (pronounced "ill-E-ak-us"). As these muscles become shorter, they lose their ability to produce optimum force, which is a major problem for cyclists, because the psoas and iliacus are the only two hip flexors capable of bringing the knee above 90 degrees. When this situation happens, the body sends in other muscles to get the job done. The problem at this point is that the other three hip flexors can't really lift the knee above 90 degrees; they can only "throw" it up there with momentum. Of the three remaining hip flexor muscles that try to compensate for the psoas and iliacus, the one that typically gets worked the hardest in cyclists is the tensor fasciae latae, or TFL. As the TFL is forced to work harder and harder to compensate for the psoas and iliacus, it begins to inflame and become irritated. The end result is chronic pain in the hip flexor region. This can all be avoided by keeping the psoas and iliacus healthy and strong by following the type of core strengthening routines found in this book.

KNEE PAIN

According to a 2010 study published in *The American Journal of Sports Medicine*, the most highly reported time-loss injury among professional road cyclists was knee pain. But don't worry, you can get knee pain as an amateur cyclist as well: A review of literature in *The Physician and Sports Medicine* estimates that 42 percent of recreational cyclists experience knee pain.

TOMMY'S TAKE   I've been very lucky in my cycling career when it comes to hip flexor pain. For whatever reason, I don't really get pain in that area. However, I still work hard to keep my psoas healthy and strong, because I've seen it become a debilitating problem for many other riders. This is yet another reason why I'm such a believer in maintaining a strong, functional core at all times—I have to keep those injuries at bay so I can focus on being fast!

Knees are located a fair distance from the core, of course, so you may wonder why chronic knee pain is being discussed in a book about core strength training. How could they possibly be related? Well, it turns out that knee pain is frequently the end result of a series of muscular imbalances that begin in the core. We can understand these more thoroughly by looking at the two most commonly reported knee injuries in cyclists: patellofemoral pain (PFP) syndrome and iliotibial band (ITB) syndrome.

"Patellofemoral pain" is a broad term used to describe pain in the front of the knee. The name "patellofemoral" describes the junction of the patella (kneecap) and the femur (thigh bone). Ironically, this pain is also referred to as "runner's knee," and one of the common treatments suggested for runners is to switch to cycling to reduce impact on the knee joint. But we all know the hidden truth about cycling: It can cause just as much knee pain as that evil high-impact stuff.

In addition to the front of the knee, the lateral, or outer, part of the knee is also a frequent pain site for cyclists. When pain is located on the lateral part of the knee or thigh, it is often because of ITB syndrome. The iliotibial band is a length of connective tissue that runs from the hip (the iliac crest) to the shinbone (the tibia). Along the way, the band passes over two bumps. One is a bony projection on the outside of your knee, called Gerdy's tubercle. The other is a bump on the hip, which has no name. The band rides over the bumps every time you bend and straighten your leg. If your ITB is tight, or if it is overworked (see below), it rubs on the bumps, gets irritated, and causes a sharp pain on the outside of your knee or hip. Often, the pain doesn't start until you're a little way into your ride.

If you are experiencing symptoms of either PFP or ITB syndrome, the first order of business is to make sure you have a proper bike fit. Sometimes adjusting

TOMMY'S TAKE

At the beginning of my training season in 2012, I was experiencing some anterior knee pain. After a few visits to the massage therapist, we tracked it to a tight psoas and a lazy gluteus medius. With a combination of massage to loosen up the tight muscles and core exercises to strengthen them, the knee pain went away and hasn't been back since.

FIGURE 2.5 **MUSCULAR IMBALANCES LEADING TO ITB AND PFP SYNDROMES**

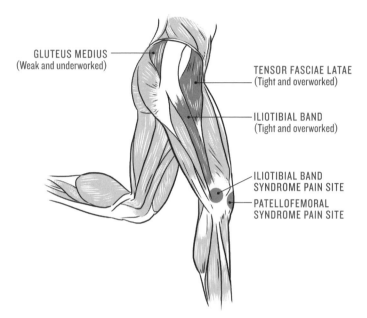

GLUTEUS MEDIUS
(Weak and underworked)

TENSOR FASCIAE LATAE
(Tight and overworked)

ILIOTIBIAL BAND
(Tight and overworked)

ILIOTIBIAL BAND
SYNDROME PAIN SITE

PATELLOFEMORAL
SYNDROME PAIN SITE

your bike's seat height can make the pain disappear in seconds. If, however, your bike fit is solid and you are still feeling chronic pain in either your knees or the lateral part of your thigh, it's time to examine muscular imbalances as the root of your pain.

A common approach that cyclists take for treating knee pain is to (a) ice the area, (b) take a lot of ibuprofen, and (c) be confused about why the pain isn't magically going away. The reason the knee pain isn't going away is that the knee isn't the problem at all; it may be the site of the pain but it is not the source of the pain. This situation is much like what happens when you walk a dog that likes to pull on the leash. The dog pulls on the end of the leash that is 5 feet away, and you consequently feel pain in the wrist that the leash is wrapped around. In order to alleviate the pain in your wrist (pain site) you must get the dog on the other end to stop pulling (pain source).

In the case of PFP and ITB syndromes, the leash is your iliotibial band, and the dog is your tensor fasciae latae (TFL). The tightness and pulling originate at the TFL, which in turn pulls on the top of the iliotibial (IT) band and causes the entire band to become irritated and overstretched. The pulling continues all the way down the IT band and ends up at the knee. Although you feel the pain in your knee, it's not the actual source of the problem; it's just the place where the pain shows up (Figure 2.5).

In order to get the TFL to stop pulling on the IT band, we have to examine the reason why the TFL is pulling in the first place. In the previous section about hip flexor pain, we learned that a common reason muscles pull and tighten up is because they are being overworked. With hip flexor pain, the TFL is overworked because it is doing the job of a tight and weak iliopsoas complex. With knee pain, the TFL is overworked because it is being forced to step in for the gluteus medius. When the gluteus medius becomes tight and weak, it loses efficiency and is unable to perform the job of stabilizing the hips. In other words, the length-tension relationship of the gluteus medius has been altered (Figure 2.4), and now a different, less-efficient muscle must step in to do the job of hip stabilization. Because the TFL is connected to the iliotibial band, it causes tightness and pulling on the IT band, which is transmitted all the way down the outside of the thigh and eventually causes knee pain on the other end.

The best approach to alleviating chronic knee pain, therefore, is to get the gluteus medius functioning properly through the use of core strengthening exercises, thereby enabling it to stabilize the hips without asking for help from the TFL.

NECK AND UPPER-BACK PAIN

Has cycling given you a brontosaurus neck? An unfortunate consequence of the optimum aerodynamic riding position is that it causes hyperextension of the neck and rounding of the upper back. End result? Brontosaurus neck. As loveable as these Jurassic herbivores are, we as humans weren't designed to have excessively long necks. In fact, a human neck that is constantly hyperextended is very problematic, mainly because it causes chronic pain in the upper back and neck.

The type of pain cyclists experience in the neck and upper back is usually described as "knots." Although it may feel like a big, hard knot, the technical term is "trigger point." These areas are extremely sensitive, and when pressure is placed on them, pain will typically shoot out (hence the name "trigger point"). Trigger points are almost

FIGURE 2.6 TRIGGER POINTS IN THE UPPER BACK AND NECK

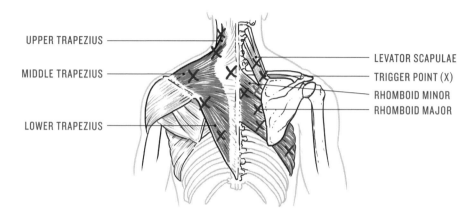

always located in the upper back, with the majority being found on the rhomboids and upper trapezius (trap) muscles (Figure 2.6). It's no coincidence that these are also the two muscles that incur the greatest amount of lengthening when you're riding.

As the rhomboids and upper traps are stretched and held at their maximum length for extended periods of time, they begin to fight back against this pull, resembling an intense game of tug-of-war. The end result is little areas of hyper-agitated tissue that typically develop along the inside edges of the shoulder blades and the back of the neck.

These localized points of pain can often create the sensation that the upper back is tight, which in turn generates the urge to stretch the area in order to alleviate the pain. Although stretching the upper back may provide temporary relief, it will exacerbate the underlying problem. The reason these trigger points occur is

TOMMY'S TAKE When I first started road cycling at a pro level, I had all kinds of sharp pain in my upper back and neck. It was always exacerbated when racing, because during races I would tense up. After a race I could barely turn my head to the side, because my neck and upper back were so riddled with trigger points. It wasn't until 2008 when I got on a good core program with Allison that all that pain in my upper back went away. Now I rarely, if ever, have those trigger points.

because the muscles of the neck and upper back are excessively overstretched and lengthened during cycling, so stretching them even more when you get off the bike is not a good idea.

Cycling puts a very specific—and very negative—strain on the muscles of the neck and upper back. Almost everyone today already suffers from rounded shoulders and a forward head carriage, thanks to the excessive number of hours we spend staring at computer screens, phones, and tablets, but cycling takes this rounding of the upper body to a new level. When you are riding, the muscles on the front side of the body contract and shorten in order to pull your shoulders forward and give you a nicely rounded back over which air can smoothly pass. If the cervical spine (neck) follows the roundedness of the thoracic spine (upper back) then your chin drops toward your chest, and you end up looking straight down at the road while you're riding. Most cyclists prefer to be looking forward when riding (highly recommended), and in order to bring the eyes up but keep the shoulders aerodynamically rounded, the body has to extend the neck out, lift the chin slightly, and crunch the back of the neck. Ouch, not comfortable. And don't forget that the neck is doing all this with the extra weight of a helmet strapped on the head above it.

When this brontosaurus-type neck position is maintained for an extended period of time, the length-tension relationship of the muscles in the upper back and neck begins to change. The muscles on the front side of the upper body become shortened, while the muscles on the back side of the upper body become lengthened (Figure 2.7). We can see from Figure 2.3 that if the resting length of a muscle is either too short or too long, the ability of that muscle to generate optimum force is drastically reduced. The end result is that no single muscle is functioning optimally, which means that the cervical and thoracic spine are not being properly supported, putting that entire area at greater risk for injury.

Trigger points create the false sensation that the area where they are located is tight, when in fact that area is overstretched. In order to relieve the pull placed on each end of the muscles of the upper back, you must release the pull that is being placed on the area by stretching the muscles on the front side of the body, which in turn causes the muscles on the back side of the muscle to contract and shorten. The

FIGURE 2.7 CHRONICALLY TIGHT MUSCLES ON THE FRONT SIDE OF THE BODY

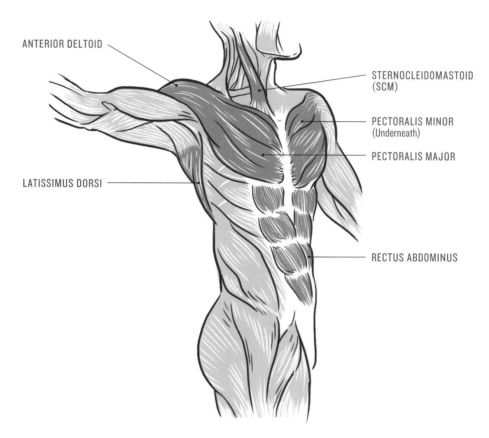

ANTERIOR DELTOID

STERNOCLEIDOMASTOID
(SCM)

PECTORALIS MINOR
(Underneath)

PECTORALIS MAJOR

LATISSIMUS DORSI

RECTUS ABDOMINUS

primary goal is to return the muscles of the neck and upper back to their optimum length-tension relationship; in order to do this, the muscles on the front side of the body must be lengthened, specifically the pectoralis major and minor, the anterior deltoid, the rectus abdominis, the sternocleidomastoid muscle (SCM), and the latissimus dorsi (Figure 2.7). Most people think of the lats as a back muscle, which is where the majority of this muscle mass is located. However, the lats insert into the front part of the shoulder blade and upper groove of the humerus (upper arm bone), and when they become tight they contribute to chronic roundedness in the upper back and neck.

Again, the trigger points will create the false sensation that the area where they are located is tight, when in fact that area is overstretched. Fight the urge to stretch your upper back if you feel trigger points after a ride!

Low-Back Pain

Low-back pain is so common that doctors simply refer to it as LBP. It is estimated that 70 to 85 percent of Americans will suffer from low-back pain at some point in their lives, and this number seems to be on the rise. Though some people are lucky enough to have a brief bout with LBP, most cases are chronic and require extensive medical treatment, dangerous prescriptions for painkillers, and sometimes surgery. Bottom line: Low-back pain is no joke, and as a cyclist you are at great risk of experiencing it.

A 2010 review of literature by the *International Sports Medicine Journal* found that low-back pain is reported by up to 60 percent of cyclists. That means as a cyclist, you have a better than even chance of experiencing low-back pain. Low-back pain is also the number one-reported reason for lost time on the bike. Your odds of experi-

TOMMY'S TAKE

Low-back pain has always been a limiter in my cycling career—I've had to drop out of races because of it, and I've missed a lot of valuable training as well. In the past, I did random core exercises and still had back pain, particularly in the sacroiliac area (the SI joint is the junction between the sacrum and the ilium; see Figure 2.8), that shot down my legs. Ever since following the routines you see in this book, I have completely eliminated all low-back pain. I don't have to slow down in races or training because of pain in my low back, which is something that most cyclists can't say.

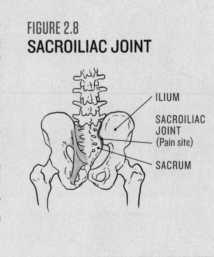

FIGURE 2.8
SACROILIAC JOINT

ILIUM

SACROILIAC JOINT
(Pain site)

SACRUM

FIGURE 2.9 **MUSCULAR IMBALANCES ASSOCIATED WITH POSTERIOR PELVIC TILT**

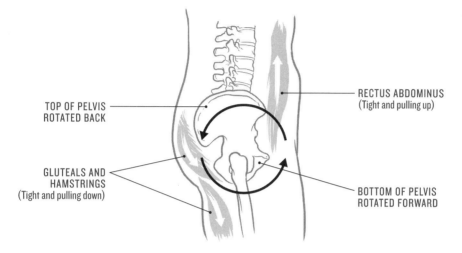

TOP OF PELVIS
ROTATED BACK

RECTUS ABDOMINUS
(Tight and pulling up)

GLUTEALS AND
HAMSTRINGS
(Tight and pulling down)

BOTTOM OF PELVIS
ROTATED FORWARD

encing low-back pain as a result of riding go up substantially if you ride more than 160 km (100 miles) per week, so the easy answer is to ride less. But then you would also have to either eat less or find a different sport, neither of which is appealing. The other option is to keep riding, but to simultaneously keep the muscles of the core strong and healthy so that the vertebrae in your low back are supported.

By now you have probably realized that almost all muscular overuse injuries stem from certain muscles being tight and overactive while others are lengthened and weak, which causes altered length-tension relationships in both sets of muscles. We have already seen how this is the root of knee pain, hip flexor pain, and upper-back and neck pain. Low-back pain is also caused by muscles working too hard or not enough, but it differs from the other overuse injuries in that the root of the problem could be a pelvis that is tilted either too far forward or too far backward. With the other injuries, the culprit is usually quite clear, which makes both diagnosis and correction fairly straightforward. With low-back pain, we have to figure out whether the pelvis is stuck in a posterior position (tailbone tucked under) or if the tilt is anterior (swayback).

When the pelvis is held in a posterior tilt, the length-tension relationships of the muscles attached to it become altered (Figure 2.9). In the case of a posterior tilt, the hamstrings, gluteals, rectus abdominis, transversus abdominis, serratus anterior, and trapezius all become tight and overactive. At the same time, the quadriceps, hip adductors, erector spinae, and rhomboids all become lengthened and weak. As we know from previous sections, the more time a muscle spends in a lengthened or shortened position, the higher the chances that it will eventually lose its ability to return to its original length. The end result is that your posture may be permanently altered, leading to a host of additional problems (see Chapter 3 for an extended discussion of this topic).

The other frequent cause of low-back pain is an excessive anterior pelvic tilt. A healthy, or neutral, pelvis has a natural anterior tilt, which is why we use the term "excessive" in this discussion. A normal anterior pelvic tilt for men is between 4 and 7 degrees and for women between 7 and 10 degrees. Often referred to as "swayback," an excessive anterior tilt in the pelvis is associated with tight quadriceps, hip flexors, erector spinae, and multifidus muscles (Figure 2.10). The lengthened and weakened

FIGURE 2.10 MUSCULAR IMBALANCES ASSOCIATED WITH ANTERIOR PELVIC TILT

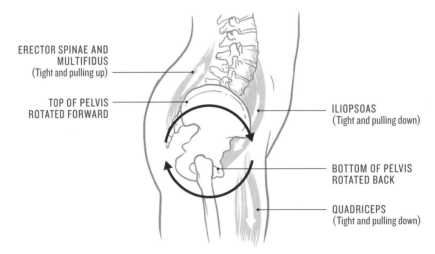

ERECTOR SPINAE AND
MULTIFIDUS
(Tight and pulling up)

TOP OF PELVIS
ROTATED FORWARD

ILIOPSOAS
(Tight and pulling down)

BOTTOM OF PELVIS
ROTATED BACK

QUADRICEPS
(Tight and pulling down)

muscles in this scenario are the rectus abdominis, external obliques, transversus abdominis, hamstrings, and gluteals. Because the hip flexors and quadriceps are shortened, cyclists with an anterior pelvis tilt often experience chronic hip flexor pain along with low-back pain.

Regardless of whether the pelvis is excessively tilted anteriorly or posteriorly, the two muscles that consistently present themselves as the most problematic are the transversus abdominis (TVA) and the glute max. Neither of these muscles is considered a low-back muscle, but when the TVA and glute max are weak, pain will often occur in the low-back area. This is yet another example of the difference between pain site and pain source; the TVA and glute max are the source of the pain, but the low back is the actual location of the pain. It all has to do with the order in which the muscles are supposed to activate to provide stabilization to the lumbar spine. In a healthy subject, the TVA should fire a fraction of a second before any movement takes place in the limbs. If the TVA doesn't fire, the pelvis and lumbar spine are not properly stabilized during movement, and the low back is allowed to move around too much, which stresses the muscles of that area and eventually causes chronic pain.

Countless studies have shown a direct correlation between low-back pain and a delayed firing of the TVA. In a 1996 article published in *Spine* magazine, Hodges and Richardson show that test subjects who experience low-back pain also have inefficient stabilization of the lumbar spine due to inactivity in the TVA. The study highlights the importance of maintaining strong, efficient core musculature to avoid pain and injury in the spine.

A delayed firing response in the TVA tends to be associated with delayed firing in the glute max as well. The primary job of the glute max is to extend the hip, which happens in cycling every time you push down on the pedal. If the glute max isn't providing enough force to extend the hip, the muscles of the low back will frequently step in and try to perform the job. This is bad news for the low-back muscles, because they will quickly become fatigued, overworked, and irritated—the perfect recipe for chronic low-back pain.

SPINAL DISC INJURIES

Disc injuries take low-back pain to a new level of seriousness. Surgery, months of rehab, and possibly even disc replacement are all common treatments for an injured disc. While some disc injuries are caused by a cycling accident, most are the end result of a long series of events that initially began with muscular imbalances in the core.

It's hard to believe that a simple muscular imbalance could eventually lead to an injured spinal disc, but this scenario plays itself out countless times with cyclists. We have already seen how muscular imbalances can lead to poor performance and muscular overuse injuries, but the importance of maintaining a strong and healthy core doesn't stop there. Besides increasing power and speed on the bike, core muscles provide the crucial service to cyclists of protecting the spine from damaging forces. These damaging forces appear in many ways, the most relevant of which is the repetitive force that cycling posture places on the lumbar spine. Without the protective armor of a strong core musculature, the spinal discs are allowed to extend and flex excessively, eventually causing the intervertebral discs to become damaged.

TOMMY'S TAKE Glute activation is not really on cycling's radar, because we generally think of the prime movers as hamstrings, quads, and calves. After all, those are the muscles that develop the most as you train. But the glutes have been a critical component in my ability to use both legs equally. Strong glutes have also helped me avoid chronic low-back pain.

I learned the importance of glute strength the hard way by injuring my low back in late 2007. Luckily, that's when I started training with Allison, and the first thing she noticed was that my glutes weren't really firing. Because they weren't firing, I was kind of a wet noodle on the bike—my spine and pelvis were flopping all over the place, and that movement was causing injury in my low back. Strengthening the connection between my low back, glutes, and hamstrings has not only alleviated my back pain but has given me a smoother pedal stroke and enabled me to be much stronger and more efficient out of the saddle.

Understanding the complexity of how a disc injury evolves is central to being able to keep the discs healthy. The journey toward unraveling this complexity must begin with the structure that houses our delicate discs: the spinal column.

COMPOSITION AND FUNCTION OF THE SPINAL COLUMN

The spinal column provides support and stability for all the extremities (arms and legs) of the body, and it houses and protects the spinal cord and all the spinal nerves. The spinal cord is like a direct telephone line from the brain to the muscles. Each pedal stroke you make starts with a thought in the brain. This thought is then transferred through the spinal cord to the muscles and tells them to complete the pedal stroke. If the alignment and function of the spinal column are compromised, the speed at which this message travels from the brain to the muscles will also be impaired, thus resulting in suboptimal muscular performance.

After years of being in the saddle, you may feel like the action of pedaling is something that happens automatically and without thought. The reality is that these pedal strokes are made possible by a series of messages sent from the brain to the muscles through a system of nerves; the signal-sending process is called "innervation." Each of our muscles has an innervation point that originates at a vertebra of the spine. Figure 2.11 illustrates which area of the spine (cervical, thoracic, lumbar, or sacrum) as well as which specific vertebra (1, 2, 3, etc.) is the home for the nerves that control the major muscles of the body. For example, the quadriceps muscles are innervated at L2 (lumbar spine, second vertebra), which means that if the second vertebra of the lumbar spine is injured, impaired, or not in its optimal alignment, it could affect the efficiency with which you are able to activate your quadriceps—clearly not an ideal situation for a cyclist. To truly understand the importance of innervation, think about what happens when the spinal nerve can no longer communicate with the muscles on the other end. All the muscles that are innervated from that point downward will not be able to function, rendering those muscles paralyzed.

The good news is that the spinal column acts as a hard protective armor for the fragile spinal cord and all the nerves that are inside. In fact, the human body is well designed to provide a safeguard for your spinal cord; not only is the spinal

FIGURE 2.11 **NERVES OF THE SPINAL COLUMN AND THE MUSCLES THEY CONTROL**

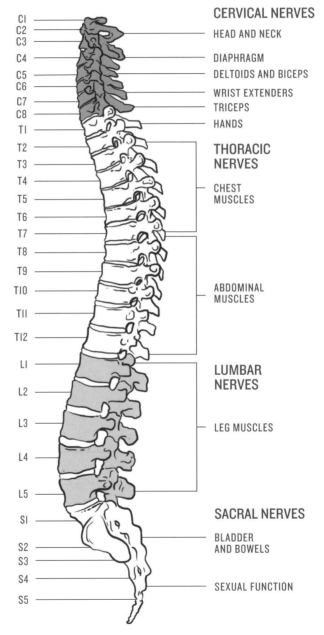

FIGURE 2.12 **HEALTHY INTERVERTEBRAL DISC**

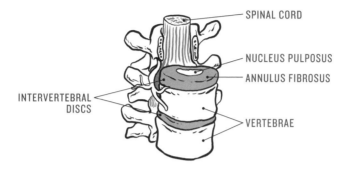

cord surrounded by the hard bones of the vertebrae, it also has padding between each vertebra called intervertebral discs. These discs are located between the 26 articulating vertebrae of the cervical, thoracic, and lumbar spinal regions. We also have 9 more fused vertebrae in the sacrum and coccyx, but they aren't separated by intervertebral discs.

The typical disc is about an inch in diameter and a quarter-inch thick, and it is composed of two parts: the nucleus pulposus and the annulus fibrosus. The nucleus pulposus is a gel-like sac in the middle of the disc that helps absorb shock and distribute force (Figure 2.12). Surrounding the nucleus pulposus is tissue called annulus fibrosus, which keeps the nucleus pulposus from leaking out and pressing against the nerves that run up and down the spinal cord.

You can think of intervertebral discs like jelly donuts—all the dough on the outside provides a neat little house for the jelly. Now imagine a stack of jelly donuts 26 high that is constantly being jostled, flexed, twisted, and contorted. If you put too much pressure on either side of the donut stack (like being in a flexed position on the bike for long periods of time), the jelly will start to squeeze out the side, which is how a disc injury is born. The reason a disc injury is so painful is not because of the leaking gel from the center of the disc, but rather because of what the gel pushes against: nerve roots. Pressure on a nerve root can cause debilitating pain that can follow the entire length of the nerve, sometimes running all the way down the back of the leg.

FIGURE 2.13 **LUMBAR VERTEBRAE AND SACRUM**

FIGURE 2.14 **STAGES OF DISC HERNIATION**

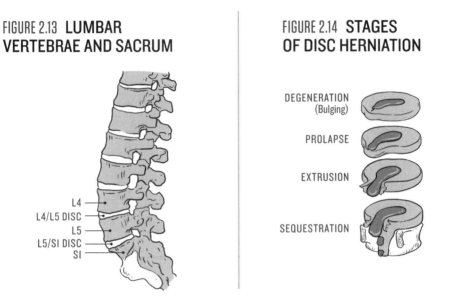

COMMON DISC INJURIES IN CYCLISTS

Almost 90 percent of disc injuries occur in the lumbar spine, most frequently between L4 and L5 and L5 and S1 (Figure 2.13). These two segments of the spine bear the most body weight, which makes them the most susceptible to injury, and they are also the areas subject to the most flexion and extension during cycling. When the L5-S1 disc is injured, it frequently puts pressure on the sciatic nerve and causes a condition known as "sciatica." When the sciatic nerve is compressed, it causes pain in the buttock (almost always on one side only) that can run all the way down the back of the leg into the calf. Cycling will often irritate sciatic nerve pain, because flexion in the L5-S1 area—which happens every time the knee moves toward the chest in a pedal stroke—is known to increase pressure on the sciatic nerve.

Sacroiliac joint pain (SI joint) is also common in cyclists. The terms "sciatica" and "SI joint pain" are often used interchangeably to refer to pain that exists in the lower back and off to one side. However, the SI joints can technically be compromised or dysfunctional without pinching the sciatic nerve. The SI joints are the junction at which the fused vertebrae of the sacrum connect with the right and left iliac bones (Figure 2.8). This is an important junction, because it connects the spine to the pelvis. When functioning correctly, there should be fewer than 4 degrees of motion and 2 mm of translation at these joints; the "translation" of a joint refers to linear movement along an axis, either side-to-side or front to back. If there is too little or too much movement in these joints, you can experience pain in the low back, the back of the hips, and even the groin and thighs. SI joint pain is notoriously persistent, but one of the best ways to prevent it is by keeping the core muscles of the low back and hips strong, so that the joints are encouraged to move properly.

If you do have the misfortune of experiencing a disc injury, you may notice that several different terms get thrown around to describe your injury. Terminology and classification of disc injuries can be confusing, as there seems to be no general consensus on the issue. One doctor may diagnose a "disc herniation," while another will call it "degeneration," and yet another will classify it as a "disc prolapse." All of these terms refer to a specific stage or level of disc injury, with degeneration (also called bulging) being the least serious and a disc sequestration being the most advanced (Figure 2.14).

The progression of a disc injury from degeneration to sequestration can take years, or it can happen practically overnight. A disc bulge can usually be treated without surgery if it is detected early enough, but once a disc reaches extrusion or sequestration there are few options besides going under the knife or learning to live with chronic pain.

One of the major determining influences in how quickly an injury progresses is the general health of the disc. Factors that contribute to disc health include age, genetics, posture, and muscle tone. Nothing can be done about the first two in this list; we all age, and we all have genetic tendencies. Posture and muscle tone, on the other hand, are well within our ability to control and improve. The most effective way to improve your posture and muscle tone around the spine is to keep the musculature of the core healthy and strong. This will allow the spine to return to its optimum position when you get off the bike and to withstand the deleterious forces of riding that are placed on the spine when you are on the bike.

Avoiding Injury

Table 2.1 summarizes the muscular overuse injuries discussed in this chapter, along with the muscular imbalances that trigger them. The most effective way to recover from or avoid these injuries is to make sure all muscles are at the correct length and can produce optimal force. A dynamic stretching routine will get the muscles to their correct length, and a functional core strength routine will ensure that they are producing enough force. All of the routines in this book contain dynamic stretching followed by functional core exercises.

In Part II you will find three different core strength programs called "Injury Prevention" that are specifically designed to decrease your chances of sustaining the injuries discussed in this chapter. The exercises in those workouts will correct the muscular weaknesses and imbalances that frequently lead to overuse injuries, thereby decreasing the amount of time you spend running to the doctor,

TABLE 2.1 SOURCES OF CHRONIC PAIN

LOCATION OF PAIN	MUSCLE(S) THAT ARE SHORTENED/LENGTHENED AND WEAK	MUSCLE(S) THAT ARE OVERACTIVE AND DOMINANT
HIP FLEXOR	Psoas, Iliacus	Tensor fasciae latae (TFL), Sartorius, Rectus femoris
KNEE (patellofemoral syndrome, iliotibial band syndrome)	Glute medius	TFL, Iliotibial band
LOW BACK	Transversus abdominis Gluteal complex	Erector spinae, Multifidus
UPPER BACK AND NECK	Rhomboids, Upper trapezius	Pectoralis major and minor, Anterior deltoid, Sternocleidomastoid

TOMMY'S TAKE I know what you're thinking: Enough talk about how to prevent injuries, what about rehabbing from injuries I get from a
crash? As hard as you try to avoid crashes, if you ride your bike enough it will happen.
Stage 6 of the 2012 Tour de France is a perfect example of this.

To say that it was a "horrific crash" is definitely an understatement. Yes, it was a
crash that I felt physically, but it was also my Tour de France dreams crashing down
around me, all the sacrifices I had made since November 2011—all the training, the
dieting, the traveling, everything went poof in about 2 seconds.

I had already crashed in stage 3 and separated my right shoulder, but the X-rays
had come back negative for a break, and I thought that if I just taped it up and took a lot
of aspirin, I might be able to ride through my recovery and do something toward the end
of the Tour. Well, stage 6 had other ideas in mind for me.

Every cyclist has a little voice in the back of his or her head that says, "If you go down
now, that's it." Usually that voice kicks in when I'm doing 50 mph on a winding downhill,
but during stage 6 of the Tour in 2012, that voice kicked in when I was already flying
through the air. Almost 90 riders went down that day, and I actually consider myself one
of the lucky ones. There were so many injured riders that there literally weren't enough
ambulances to take us all to the local hospitals. I sat in the back of a car on the side of
the road for 3 hours before I was finally transported to the emergency room.

Amazingly, I didn't have any broken bones, but I did separate my other shoulder.
I also had 8 hematomas, and both sides of my body were covered in road rash, bruises,
and bone bruises.

I spent the next three nights in a hospital near Charles de Gaulle Airport in Paris,
waiting for the swelling to go down enough to allow me to fly home. I passed the time
by watching the Tour on TV—not exactly the way I thought I'd be seeing the finish line!
During those three days I had a lot of time to start thinking about how I was going to
recover and get ready for the USA Pro Challenge in my home state of Colorado. I knew
I was going to have lots of work to do when I got home.

Luckily, I was able to start riding again after about two weeks. I had developed
all kinds of complicated muscular imbalances from my injuries, and I started pedaling
weird because I was favoring my right leg. Allison had me do lots of glute activation
exercises, trying to get my hips working evenly.

My upper back was also a wreck and had lots of painful knots, because my
shoulders were in a frozen position, so I had to work really hard on getting mobility in
my thoracic spine. That was probably the most challenging part of rehab. I can't even
count how many sets of Shoulder Blade Squeezes I did (see the Level I exercises). No

Continued on next page »

Continued from previous page

one wants to go back to a Level I routine in the middle of the season, but it had to be done. I was aware from previous injuries that it's never just the site of the injury that suffers; injuries create a domino effect of problems.

So I gave everything I had and was really smart about not overtraining. Instead I focused on training smart, and a big part of that was making sure my core muscles were strong enough to support me.

There was no way that core strength could have gotten me out of that stage 6 crash, but it sure did help me recover from the crash more quickly. After only a few months of working on injury routines, I was right back up to my favorite routine: Tommy D's Optimum Performance Workout! In fact, we did the photo shoot for the exercise section of this book just a little more than two months after the Tour de France crash. This stuff really works!

the chiropractor, the acupuncturist, and the pharmacy. By keeping your core healthy and strong, you will be able to enjoy pain-free cycling and concentrate on the important things, like increasing your power output!

CHAPTER 3

Posture

Cyclists and correct posture have always had a contentious relationship. Correct posture calls for the body to be in optimal structural alignment—chest lifted, shoulder blades flat against the back, and pelvis in a neutral position. But for cyclists to achieve an effective aerodynamic position on the bike, they need to have a rounded back, caved-in shoulders, and a neck that is cranked down and forward. In other words, good cycling demands bad posture. Our mothers and first-grade teachers are sucking in their breath with horror right now.

It is indisputable that cyclists who ride with a rounded back are more aerodynamic. Logic would therefore dictate that everyone who wants to be a good cyclist should work on developing an excessively rounded back. While this argument may seem plausible at first glance, it fails to consider the larger picture of why good posture is important not only for cycling performance but also for long-term good health. Correct posture is essential for cyclists because it reduces the risk of spinal injuries and helps decrease the low-back and shoulder pain that come with endless hours in the saddle. Correct posture also helps to increase proper breathing technique, which is essential when you're pushing the limits of your anaerobic zone, climbing steep inclines, or out-sprinting your competition to the finish line.

Off the bike, good posture helps reduce the occurrence of headaches, staves off bone density loss, and decreases the likelihood of developing ischemic tissue buildup (blood-starved muscle). And let's not forget the confidence and demand for respect that are associated with good posture. All of these benefits will be discussed in detail throughout this chapter, beginning with a basic discussion of the difference between static and dynamic posture.

Static Posture

The spinal column is meant to be highly flexible. It is capable of bending, twisting, rotating, and then returning to a neutral position, all without sustaining any long-term damage. This neutral position is called "static posture," and it refers to the position of the spinal column when it's at rest. In its proper static alignment, the spine exhibits natural curves that flex forward and backward as shown in Figure 3.1.

The cervical and lumbar regions of the spine should exhibit slight lordosis, which is a curve that is convex anteriorly (to the front) and concave posteriorly (to the rear). In a static position, the cervical spine should have a 30- to 35-degree lordotic curve, and the lumbar spine should have a 45-degree lordotic curve.

In contrast to the cervical and lumbar regions, the thoracic and sacral regions of the spinal column should exhibit a curve that is concave anteriorly and convex posteriorly. This type of curve is called kyphosis. A healthy thoracic spine will have a 40-degree kyphotic curve, and a healthy sacral spine will have a 65-degree kyphotic curve. These numbers represent an average, and they can vary from person to person.

TOMMY'S TAKE Breathing well has always been my trump card. I have a small frame, but somehow I have this enormous barrel chest sitting right in the middle of it. With naturally large lungs, I guess I was destined to be a cyclist. Genetics may have given me a big chest, but it's up to me to make sure I don't collapse my chest cavity while I'm riding. I can always tell when I'm being lazy about my posture on the bike: My breathing feels restricted, and I can't access all my lung capacity on climbs.

FIGURE 3.1 **NATURAL CURVES AND REGIONS OF THE SPINE**

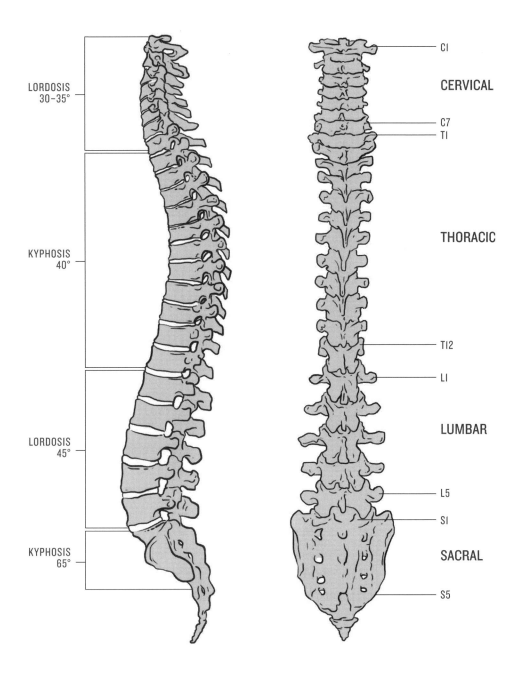

LORDOSIS
30–35°

KYPHOSIS
40°

LORDOSIS
45°

KYPHOSIS
65°

CI

CERVICAL

C7
TI

THORACIC

TI2

LI

LUMBAR

L5

SI

SACRAL

S5

TOMMY'S TAKE   The proper posture when descending is to keep your body as relaxed as possible. Your arms and legs should be supple, but your core should be engaged in order to keep your center of gravity stable over the bike. This will allow you to navigate turns and to react to any debris and bumps that you might ride over.

For example, the curves of a newborn's spine are not fully cemented, and they will change as the child grows. Another typical variation is that women tend to exhibit a greater degree of lumbar lordosis than men.

Regardless of these variations, the key lesson to be learned about static posture is that the curvature in one region of the spine affects the curvature in other regions. In other words, if the curvature of the cervical region of your spine is incorrect, the curvatures in other regions of your spine will change in order to compensate. By allowing one region of your spine to exhibit improper alignment, you are allowing the first domino to be tipped, which is a situation that can eventually result in injury, decreased neuromuscular function, and poor performance on the bike.

Dynamic Posture

To your mother, posture meant standing up straight, but in fact "posture" can refer to the position of the body in motion as well as the position of the body at rest. Posture is therefore both static (at rest) and dynamic (in motion). When you are on your bike, your body employs both static and dynamic posture for balance and control.

Cycling is a unique sport, in that the body is constantly in motion, yet in order to be stable and have control of the bike, the body must also be still. You could see this vividly if you caught the video of the nerve-wracking descent down the Col du Tourmalet in stage 16 of the 2011 Tour de France. Despite the writhing curves, rough pavement, and breakneck speed, the riders strung out in a long line were almost completely still aboard their bikes as they worked their way to the valley. Their near-motionless position on their bikes is a perfect example of static yet dynamic posture at its finest.

Now think about the last time you went for a ride with a group of friends. You came to a stop sign and needed to turn left. As you decelerated, you turned your head to the left to check for oncoming traffic, but you kept the bike heading straight so you didn't swerve into cars or one of your friends on another bike. This simple action is an example of the importance of having a highly supple, flexible spinal column. Your cervical and thoracic spine had to perform lateral flexion (side-to-side) as well as axial rotation (twisting), while your lumbar spine worked to remain as stable as possible so that you didn't tip over.

If any part of your spinal column has limited range of motion, you will have to move your entire body in order to accomplish the task of twisting, turning, flexing, or bending. It is possible to have a limited range of motion because of something temporary like sleeping on your neck incorrectly, but many times the spinal column has a limited range of motion as a result of improper alignment or poor posture, otherwise known as a "postural distortion."

Postural Distortions

Unfortunately, most of us do not have perfect static or dynamic posture. In fact, postural distortions (commonly known as "poor posture") have become so common that when someone with perfect posture walks by, heads turn to stare. Because of the ever-increasing use of computers, cell phones, and time spent sitting and slouching, the presence and severity of postural distortions is growing at an alarming rate. As a

TOMMY'S TAKE Over the years, I've been fitted, refitted, and fit some more on my bikes in order to find the fastest racing position. Usually the changes are adjustments of just a few millimeters, but the impact feels huge. The one thing I've learned is that the more compact I am, the faster I feel, especially on my TT bike. The closer my limbs are to my core, the more power I can generate. But being hunched up on the bike means I have to work hard to combat the cycling slouch when I'm off the bike. I do this by committing to a year-round core strengthening routine.

cyclist, you are at even greater risk of developing postural problems because of how many hours you spend bending forward on your bike.

Think about the typical progression of your day: wake up from eight hours of sleeping in a curled-up position, ride your bike in an aerodynamic position, go to work and hunch over your computer for eight hours, then go home and spend another four hours slouching on the couch. At no point during your day did you

TOMMY'S TAKE

I was on the third of four laps in a mountain bike race in Golden, Colorado, and I had a lead of more than 2 minutes. I was focused, controlled, and completely within myself, gliding my SoBe/Cannondale over the muddy terrain. About 1 kilometer from the start/finish line was a steep ascent that required staying in the saddle to maintain traction on the sloppy trail. I hit the climb and dug deep for power. Suddenly, instead of accelerating up the incline, my legs went to mush. A sharp, horrible pain appeared in my lower back, and I instantly lost the ability to pedal.

I got off my bike and pushed it to the top of the hill, thinking if I could stretch out my back, the pain would decrease. Stretch after stretch, nothing remedied my situation. The pain was so bad I couldn't even consider finishing the race; I dropped out with one lap to go.

After the race, I was sure I had just tweaked my back a tad and that a little rest would cure the problem. I took some time off, and when the pain disappeared, I jumped back on my bike as if nothing had happened. I was totally fine, until weeks later the same thing happened at another race—sharp pain in my low back, loss of muscle use in my leg. I was super frustrated because I couldn't figure out what was wrong.

I spent months seeing specialists who tried to reduce the pain by looking for an injury in the area where the pain was coming from. But the true solution came from correcting my poor posture! Yep, that "cycling slouch" had led to intense back pain. Years and years of cycling had created muscle imbalances, which showed up visibly in the form of poor posture. These muscle imbalances eventually turned into the injury in my sacroiliac (SI) joint.

The solution was to strengthen and stretch my core muscles. Before I got on the bike each day, I performed an extensive core routine (see Part II). The exercises stimulated each muscle group, so it would be functioning properly when I rode, and it helped my core get stronger at the same time. After only one month of hard work, my SI was working properly, my posture had improved, and I felt much more "solid" on the bike.

FIGURE 3.2 **PROBLEMS ASSOCIATED WITH POSTURAL DISTORTIONS**

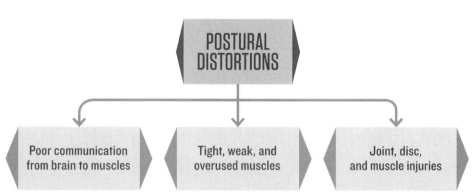

practice proper static or dynamic posture. Now take this scenario and multiply it by the number of days you have been following this routine—has it been months, years, even decades? It's easy to see how patterns of postural distortion develop slowly over time without us even realizing how much cumulative damage we are doing to our precious spinal columns.

Postural distortions are associated with several performance concerns discussed in previous chapters, including poor communication from the brain to the muscles; tight, weak, and overused muscles; and joint, disc, and muscle injuries. It's difficult to say whether these conditions are caused by postural distortions or the distortions are causing the problems, but the one thing we do know is that they are inextricably linked (Figure 3.2).

One of the many reasons postural distortions can sneak up on us is because they come in so many forms and can be difficult to recognize. By definition, a postural distortion refers to any deviation from the optimal alignment of the skeleton. Poor posture can appear at any place on the body (even your feet!) but we are going to

TOMMY'S TAKE

Lateral flexion comes in really handy when you're trying to chat with buddies on a ride, but most of the time I use my lateral spinal flexion to see how far back my competition is!

FIGURE 3.3 **EXCESSIVE CERVICAL LORDOSIS**

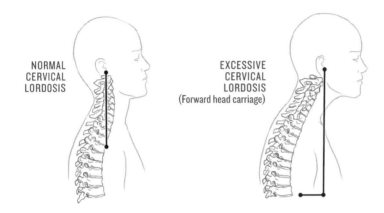

NORMAL
CERVICAL
LORDOSIS

EXCESSIVE
CERVICAL
LORDOSIS
(Forward head carriage)

FIGURE 3.4 **EXCESSIVE THORACIC KYPHOSIS**

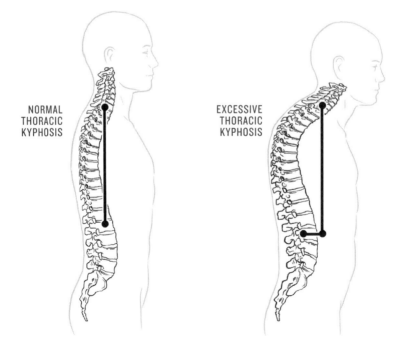

NORMAL
THORACIC
KYPHOSIS

EXCESSIVE
THORACIC
KYPHOSIS

focus on the five main types of postural distortions that are directly related to the spinal column.

EXCESSIVE CERVICAL LORDOSIS

We know from earlier in the chapter that lordosis refers to a curvature of the spine that is convex anteriorly and concave posteriorly. If the lordotic curve of the cervical spine is too great, the neck will become pushed forward so that the ears are not lined up directly above the shoulders (Figure 3.3). This type of postural distortion is also called "forward head carriage."

Excessive cervical lordosis is problematic for a variety of reasons, but the one of greatest concern is that the cervical spine is the leader of the pack; when the cervical spine moves, the rest of the body follows. If you turn your head to the left, the rest of your torso will rotate. Likewise if you extend your head too far forward on a regular basis (e.g., every time you ride), your thoracic spine will follow suit and start to curve forward, then the lumbar spine will start to abnormally curve as well. By keeping your cervical spine in healthy alignment you are doing the rest of your spine a favor.

Negative effects of excessive cervical lordosis for cyclists include the following:

> » Chronic neck pain
> » Headaches
> » Permanent forward curvature of the neck
> » Chain reaction of excessive curvature into the thoracic and lumbar areas of the spine

EXCESSIVE THORACIC KYPHOSIS

The telltale signs of an excessive thoracic curve are rounded (or protracted) shoulders and a chest that is caved in (Figure 3.4). It is extremely rare to meet someone who does not have at least a slightly exaggerated thoracic curve, and this is especially true among cyclists.

The primary reason for cyclists to cultivate a healthy thoracic spine is that it enables the chest cavity to be flexible and open, which allows the lungs to fill to capacity and then send all that oxygen to your muscles—not to mention, it allows you to fly up steep inclines without sucking air in front of your friends. If your thoracic spine is excessively rounded forward, the muscles on the front side of your body become tight and inhibited, frozen just like your mom warned you would happen if you made that face too much. If the muscles stay "frozen" for a long enough period of time, it will literally become impossible to unstick them.

Negative effects of excessive thoracic kyphosis for cyclists include the following:

- Decreased breathing capacity
- Chronic upperback pain
- Permanent curvature of the upper back

EXCESSIVE LUMBAR LORDOSIS

As mentioned before, excessive lumbar lordosis (or anterior pelvic tilt) is seen more frequently in women than in men. The dead giveaway for lumbar lordosis is a pant line or belt that sits higher in the back than in the front, which is demonstrated clearly in Figure 3.5. The top of the pelvis is tilted forward (anterior), whereas the bottom of the pelvis is tilted backward and slightly up. As a result, it may look like a person with this condition is sticking his or her bottom out in the back and belly out in the front.

Excessive lumbar lordosis carries all kinds of side effects, the most common of which is chronic lower-back pain. The vertebrae of the lumber spine are the thickest of the spinal column, and they come with the thickest intervertebral discs as well. The size of the vertebrae is a good thing in terms of protecting the lower back and pelvis and all the nerves housed inside, but as they say, "The bigger they are, the harder they fall." In other words, the bigger the vertebrae, the more potential for damage.

A great majority of disc injuries (herniation, rupture, degeneration) happen in the lumbar region, and these types of injuries can sideline you for a long time. Not only will you miss precious training time while you recover, you may also sustain permanent

FIGURE 3.5 **EXCESSIVE LUMBAR LORDOSIS**

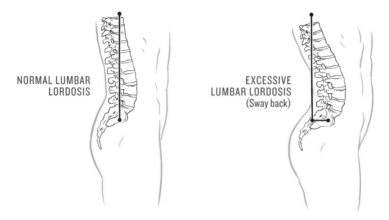

NORMAL LUMBAR
LORDOSIS

EXCESSIVE
LUMBAR LORDOSIS
(Sway back)

nerve damage in the lumbar region. The nerves of the lumbar region control the glu-teals, hamstrings, quadriceps, and calves—muscles that cyclists depend on when riding.

Negative effects of excessive lumbar lordosis for cyclists include the following:

» Chronic lower-back pain
» Injured discs
» Impaired muscle function of the legs

EXCESSIVE LUMBAR KYPHOSIS

Excessive lumbar kyphosis (or posterior pelvic tilt) is very common in cyclists, mainly because this is the position that the pelvis is in while you are riding. It is characterized by the tailbone being tucked under the body and the front of the pant line being higher than the back (Figure 3.6). For cyclists, excessive lumbar kyphosis is often coupled with excessive thoracic kyphosis in order to achieve an optimum aerodynamic position on the bike.

The same potential for disc damage that is present with excessive lumbar lordo-sis is also present with lumbar kyphosis. An additional drawback of lumbar kyphosis is that it pulls on the hamstrings and causes tightness, making it difficult to access the full power potential of the muscle.

Negative effects of excessive lumbar kyphosis for cyclists include the following:

» Chronic lower-back pain
» Injured discs
» Impaired muscle function of the legs

LATERAL PELVIC TILT

Excessive curvatures of the spine don't have to be from front to back; they can also result from the pelvis being higher on one side than the other (Figure 3.7). This type of postural distortion is more common than you may think, and it can be a major contributing factor to pain in the sacroiliac joint. If you have ever experienced sharp pain at the very bottom of your spine and a little to the side, chances

FIGURE 3.6 **EXCESSIVE LUMBAR KYPHOSIS**

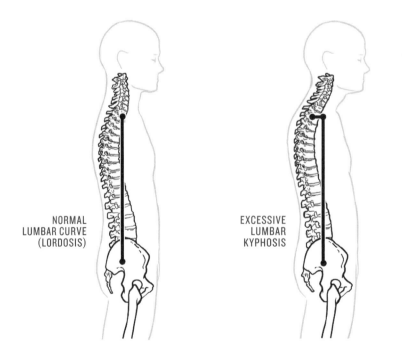

NORMAL
LUMBAR CURVE
(LORDOSIS)

EXCESSIVE
LUMBAR
KYPHOSIS

FIGURE 3.7 **LATERAL PELVIC TILT**

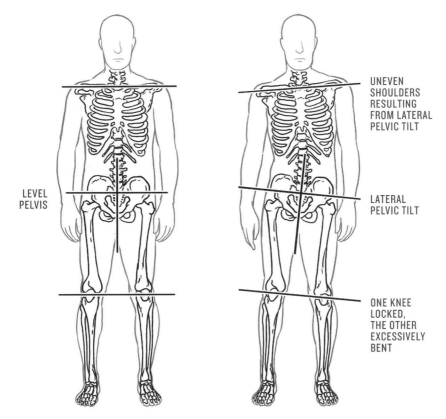

LEVEL
PELVIS

UNEVEN
SHOULDERS
RESULTING
FROM LATERAL
PELVIC TILT

LATERAL
PELVIC TILT

ONE KNEE
LOCKED,
THE OTHER
EXCESSIVELY
BENT

are you had a misalignment of the SI joint (see page 46 for a fuller discussion of SI joint injuries). This joint is the connection between the sacrum (lower part of the spine) and the ilium (part of the pelvis), and the strongest ligaments in the body can be found here.

The primary purpose of the SI joint is to enable the pelvis and spine to withstand the jolting effects of walking, running, jumping, and other activities that put stress on the body. When the SI joint is not properly aligned, the stability of the pelvis and lower spine will be compromised and the nerves in that area will become pinched. People with severe SI joint problems can experience shooting pain that runs all the way down the back of the leg to the calf.

Negative effects of lateral pelvic tilt for cyclists include the following:

⟫ Chronic SI joint pain
⟫ Permanent lateral curvature of the lower spine.

Causes of Postural Distortions

Postural distortions are sometimes caused by skeletal disorders such as cerebral palsy or scoliosis. However, these conditions are statistically rare; the more likely cause is one of the following conditions.

CONTINUOUS AND REPETITIVE POSTURAL STRESS

If you hold the previously listed postural distortions for a long period of time—which is almost always the case unless you undertake an exercise routine to correct the problems—you are causing continuous postural stress on the body. Repetitive postural stress refers to a position of the body that is assumed for a finite period of time and then changed. As discussed earlier in this chapter, cyclists usually maintain poor posture on the bike in order to increase aerodynamic efficiency.

INCORRECT AND REPETITIVE OVERUSE OF MUSCLES

This topic was discussed extensively in Chapter 1 when we looked at how muscular weakness and inefficiency can result from using your muscles incorrectly and from using the wrong muscles to perform repetitive actions. We also know from Chapter 2 that muscles become tight and restricted when they are used repetitively, causing them to pull your joints and bones into the wrong position. In other words, overusing your muscles in the wrong way can pull your spine and pelvis into the wrong position and either cause or exacerbate postural distortions.

BEING SEDENTARY

Lack of activity leads to muscular atrophy (loss of muscle mass), which is a problem because your muscles hold up your bones. Without muscles, bones and joints are left

TESTING YOUR POSTURE

With all this talk about what constitutes good posture, you probably want to know how your profile stacks up. Here are simple ways to self-diagnose your current posture situation and get a clear picture of what needs to be improved.

Signs that you have excessive **CERVICAL SPINE LORDOSIS** *(see Figure 3.3)*:
» A profile picture reveals your ears are not lined up directly above your collar bone.
» When you look up at the ceiling, the front of your neck feels extremely tight.

Signs that you have excessive **THORACIC KYPHOSIS** *(see Figure 3.4)*:
» When you lie **flat** on your back, the outer edges of your shoulder blades and the backs of your shoulders do not touch the ground.
» It is difficult to interlace your fingers behind your back, or if you can interlace them, it causes extreme pulling in the front of your shoulders and chest.

Signs that you have excessive **LUMBAR LORDOSIS** *(see Figure 3.5)*:
» When you lie **flat** on your back, you can easily slide your hand between your low back and the ground.
» The front of your belt, pants, skirt, or shorts regularly sits lower than the back.
» Your abdomen protrudes in the front, but when you squeeze your glutes and drop your tailbone down, the abdomen pulls back in.

Signs that you have excessive **LUMBAR KYPHOSIS** *(see Figure 3.6)*:
» If you stand up tall and try to arch your body backward, you feel "stuck" and can't go much past your starting point.
» Your hamstrings are extremely tight, and you have always struggled with touching your toes.

Signs that you have **LATERAL PELVIC TILT** *(see Figure 3.7)*:
» You frequently stand with all your weight on one foot.
» One side of your pant line is higher than the other.
» You experience tightness and discomfort in one side of your lower back but not on the other.

unsupported, unstable, and at greater risk for fracture and other injuries. On average, the human body loses 0.5 to 1.0 percent of muscle mass each year after the age of 25, and this mass is typically replaced with fat tissue. Loss of muscle mass can be avoided by following a regular exercise program; including core exercises in your workout routine will help keep the muscles surrounding the spine and pelvis healthy and strong.

LACK OF CORE STRENGTH

Even if you have a healthy amount of muscle mass, those muscles may not be functioning efficiently. The muscles of the core hold up your spinal column, and if those muscles aren't strong, it will be very difficult for you to correct your postural distortions.

How to Correct Your Postural Distortions

Being aware of your postural distortions is a great first step; the next step is to work on correcting them. People often feel discouraged, anxious, and self-conscious when they first discover their posture needs a little help. Take comfort in knowing that your posture can be dramatically improved with the correct exercise protocol.

In Part II of this book you will find core workout routines that help correct each one of the postural distortions discussed in this chapter. Have more than one postural

TOMMY'S TAKE

When I first started working with Allison in February 2008, my core was in pretty rough shape. I was still recovering from a nasty crash in the Vuelta a España (Tour of Spain) a few months earlier, and the bulging disc I had in my lower back was causing major pain every time I rode. Basically my whole body felt broken and weak. I remember when Allison had me do a TT Hold during our first training session so she could see what kind of shape I was in—I lasted about 10 seconds! I was frustrated and discouraged, but I knew that my core would never get stronger if I gave up and walked away.

If you struggle with some of the exercises in this book, just think about me falling on my face during a TT Hold! Then get back up and try it again, because that's how you get stronger, and that's how you reach your goals.

problem to correct? No problem—almost everyone has multiple postural concerns, so the workout routines are designed to work on several areas at the same time. As with all things in life, if you want to improve your posture, you have to be diligent and consistent in reaching your goals. The exercises in this book will help you do that.

Additional Benefits of Good Posture

Think of someone you know with picture-perfect posture. This person stands tall, proud, shoulders pulled back, head held high, and chest lifted. Do you listen when this person speaks? Does this person exude confidence and demand respect from others? If statistics are true, the answer to both of these questions is "yes." *Psychological Science* published an article in its January 2011 edition that cited three scientific studies showing that posture, not title or role, determines whether or not participants exhibited power-related behaviors. In the boardroom, power-related behaviors can mean anything from taking action to commanding an audience. Imagine if you could transfer these same behaviors to your performance on the bike.

Many cyclists erroneously believe that confidence on the bike can only come from being in great shape and logging tons of hours in the saddle so that you feel comfortable when someone is riding 2 inches off your wheel. While these two aspects are certainly important, let's not underestimate the feelings of confidence that come with being strong and secure on your bike. You know your core muscles are so rock solid that you can easily control your bike in the most unpredictable situations—you're confident, empowered, and totally in control. Can you feel your chest lifting slightly as you imagine yourself in this situation? Now imagine how tall and proud you will be standing on the podium as you receive your well-earned reward for a great race—all of which is possible thanks to your strong core and great posture.

WORKOUTS AND EXERCISES

PART II

CHAPTER 4

Flexibility

Stretching is boring. Stretching is pointless. Stretching hurts. I don't have time for stretching. I'll stretch later. Let's just start riding, and I'll loosen up.

Sound familiar? The laundry list of excuses cyclists use to get out of stretching is long, but no excuse changes the fact that achieving and maintaining optimum flexibility is essential for peak performance. Flexibility refers to the ability of the soft tissue to allow full range of motion in the joints. If your joints don't have the ability to move, your performance will plummet, because you won't be able to access the full amount of strength and power your muscles can provide. In Chapter 2, we discussed the "length-tension relationship" of muscles: If the resting length of a muscle is too long or too short, the muscles will not be able to produce peak force (Figure 2.3, page 30). Besides optimizing your power production, proper flexibility also helps reduce muscle soreness, improve posture, and decrease the amount of stress put on joints.

Before you lie down on the ground and start frantically stretching your hammies to gain more power for that group ride on Saturday, you need to know that all stretching is not the same. Not only are there multiple types of stretching, but performing the wrong type of stretching at the wrong time can actually increase your chance of injury and decrease your performance. Let's do a quick overview of the different types of stretching so that you can gain a better understanding of how each can play into performance on the bike.

Static Stretching

Static stretching is what most people think of as "stretching." Static stretching is passive and is performed by manually moving a muscle to a certain point of tension and holding it. An example of a static stretch that cyclists frequently perform is the standing quad stretch—you hold on to something with your right hand and bring your left heel to your left buttock and hold it there for a little bit, then switch sides. Then you bend over and try to reach your toes in order to stretch your hamstrings. Hold that for a few seconds and, hey, you're ready to ride! Except that by doing static stretches before you ride, you just drastically decreased the power output potential of your legs.

Over the past decade, numerous studies have emerged that suggest static stretching before exercise decreases muscular power, endurance, and balance. This holds true for performance in sports that are strength-based (weight lifting) as well as endurance-based (cycling). The evidence is so convincing that both the National

TOMMY'S TAKE In the past, I would frequently wake up the morning of a race feeling pretty productive and think it would be a good idea to do a stretching routine before the race. I made the mistake of doing static stretching, mainly because that was what I thought "stretching" was all about. I never really made the connection between static stretching and subpar performance, until Allison told me that static stretching can actually decrease performance. That's when I realized that on the days I did static stretches before a race, the first 30 to 60 minutes of that stage felt stagnant, almost like I still needed to warm up. Now I only do static stretching after I ride, and I've found that it helps me cool down and helps my muscles feel like they are relaxing and shutting off—a great benefit, but definitely not the feeling I want to have when I start my ride!

Academy of Sports Medicine and the European College of Sports Sciences have taken an official stance against static stretching before exercise. So why would anyone ever do static stretching? Although static stretching should not be performed before an athletic activity, it is effective for increasing soft tissue extensibility *after* exercise. In other words, static stretching is useful for lengthening soft tissue, which is something you want to do after you ride. Static stretching is also effective for addressing postural distortions and getting chronically tight muscles to loosen up.

When used properly, static stretching has certain benefits, and if you are not going for a ride after your core routine, then feel free to throw in some static stretches at the end of the workout. Just remember that in order to see maximum results in increasing soft tissue extensibility, static stretches should be held for a minimum of 30 seconds. A great resource is *Delavier's Stretching Anatomy* by Frederic Delavier, which gives examples of numerous static stretches with accompanying muscle diagrams.

The sample programs in this book, however, do not incorporate this form of stretching at all. This may seem odd, given the amount of coverage we gave to correcting your posture in Chapter 3. However, the programs in this book have been designed to be performed before you ride, and since static stretching before a ride decreases power and increases risk of injury, the only type of stretching we employ in these programs is dynamic stretching.

Proprioceptive Neuromuscular Facilitation

Proprioceptive neuromuscular facilitation (PNF) is a predominantly static form of stretching that requires assistance from a partner or coach to move the muscle into a stretched position. Because PNF requires the muscle to be held in a static stretch, this type of stretching has the same negative performance implications as static stretching and should not be used before a workout. Studies have shown that all variations of PNF stretching cause a significant decrease in limb velocity and movement time. For example, athletes who perform PNF stretching and then take a vertical jump test consistently see a decrease of 5 percent in jump height. Furthermore,

TOMMY'S TAKE   Being a pro cyclist definitely has some perks, and having a team of soigneurs at every race is one of them. When I'm done riding for the day (never beforehand) a soigneur will take me through a series of assisted stretches, which is painful but worth it. The quantitative effect I feel over time is that I'm actually making progress with my flexibility, whereas stretching on my own always allows me the opportunity to cut my stretching routine short or not stretch the muscles that are the tightest.

pre-exercise PNF has also been shown to decrease muscular power and endurance for up to 60 minutes after the stretch is performed.

As with static stretching, PNF stretching has also failed to produce any solid evidence confirming that it helps reduce or prevent injuries when performed before an activity. Given the depth and magnitude of scientific arguments against performing PNF stretches before activity, it should never be used as a warm-up method. However, PNF has been shown to increase joint range of motion and can be employed after a workout in order to increase range of motion.

There are three main variations of PNF stretching: hold-relax, hold-relax with agonist contraction, and contract-relax. All three variations are based on a protocol of having a partner passively move the muscle to its point of resistance, then having the athlete either push against that resistance or simply allowing the partner to hold the stretch (you can also use a strap to perform the stretch yourself, although studies have suggested this method is not as effective).

Let's use the basic supine (lying on your back) hamstring stretch to understand the differences. The athlete will typically lie on the ground or on a stretching table with one leg relaxed straight on the ground and the other leg (also being kept as straight as possible) being lifted by the partner. With the hold-relax variation, the partner gently pushes the athlete's leg up to its first point of resistance, holds it for 10 seconds, then allows the hamstring to relax before pushing it again to a second point of resistance, which should, in theory, be farther than the first point.

The hold-relax with agonist contraction starts the same way, except when the first point of resistance is reached, the athlete then gently pushes the leg back against the partner, which creates a hamstring (agonist) contraction. The partner pushes back against the athlete so that the leg remains in the same position.

In the contract-relax variation, the partner allows the athlete to slowly lower the leg to the ground by only providing gentle resistance against the leg.

Ballistic Stretching

Ballistic stretching is probably the most misunderstood and improperly used form of stretching. This type of stretching involves "bouncing" into a stretch and using a springboard-type effect to supposedly lengthen the muscles. A good example is repeatedly trying to touch your toes by bouncing up and down and trying to get farther down with each bounce.

There are several points of concern with ballistic stretching. First, by forcing a muscle or joint into an extended position, there is a significant chance of causing muscle tearing and tendon or ligament damage. In fact, most muscle tears and injuries happen in a similar way: You're out for a leisurely jog and accidently slip off the curb, causing a sudden jerking (or bouncing) motion in your leg, which results in a torn muscle in the quadriceps or hamstrings.

Second, ballistic stretching is almost always performed at the very beginning of a workout when the muscles are cold and don't have adequate blood flow. This is akin to pulling a rubber band out of a freezer and giving it a harsh tug. The band will likely snap in two, or at the very least develop multiple tears along the weakest points. Bottom line: Avoid ballistic stretching unless you're an exceptionally high-level athlete who has previously performed ballistic stretching under the supervision of a qualified coach or trainer.

Dynamic Stretching

In contrast to static stretching, dynamic stretching can and should be done before exercise. Dynamic stretching refers to the act of moving joints and muscles through their available range of motion by using muscular force and momentum. Dynamic stretches are not held; instead, the body is in continuous motion. The difference makes dynamic stretching extremely effective for preparing the body for activity, but the benefits don't stop there. The list includes the following:

» Increased muscular strength and power
» Improved length-tension relationship of muscles
» Increased range of motion
» Decreased chance of injury
» Optimization of muscle-firing patterns
» Increased blood flow to muscles

Athletes and coaches around the world are jumping on the dynamic stretching bandwagon because the evidence is essentially undeniable that it helps facilitate better athletic performance. Gone are the days of a team of football players all lying on the 50-yard line, holding a static hamstring stretch before a game. Instead, you will see these same players making their way up and down the field doing straight leg kicks, butt kicks, walking lunges, and torso twists. These are all examples of dynamic stretches, and they all work. While static stretching literally puts the muscles to

TOMMY'S TAKE In addition to my dynamic stretching routine, I have a few specific ways in which I ease into riding hard once I'm on the bike. The approaches I use vary according to whether I am doing a training ride, a stage race, or a time trial. For training rides, I warm up by doing the first 10 to 20 minutes at a high cadence with very light resistance. I try not to pay attention to my power meter, and I just listen to my body and ease into it. After about 20 minutes of this easy pedaling, I'm ready for a hard workout. In a stage race, the first 1 to 2 km is always what is called a "neutral start," which gives us all time to start spinning. A lead car takes us through the neutral zone at a slow speed, and at the end of the zone there is a red flag and sign that says "0 km," and that signals the true start to the race. At that point, I'm ready to go. To warm up for a time trial, I try to do 20 minutes of easy riding on a bike trainer, followed by a few hard efforts to open up a bit. Then I go back to some easy riding. All in all, I might spend an hour on the bike trainer warming up for a time trial.

sleep, dynamic stretching helps optimize muscle-firing patterns and increases blood flow to the muscles.

The stretches included in the core routines in this book are all dynamic stretches, and they are all performed at the beginning of the routine in order to prepare the muscles for a successful core workout. Like a lot of things that are good for you, though, they aren't the easiest things to incorporate into your exercise routine. In fact, after your first session, you might be a little sore, a little bored, and a lot surprised at your own inflexibility. Don't let this discourage you; think instead of how many times you had to ride up that climb with a 15 percent grade before you didn't feel like puking at the top.

Stretching should be as indispensable to your cycling routine as keeping your tires aired up. Just as you would never jump on your bike for a 3-hour ride without checking the tire pressure (because you know that riding with soft tires is dangerous and will slow you down), you should never voluntarily handicap yourself by skipping a stretching routine before a workout. You just need to get past the psychological barrier of immediate gratification. When you put air in your tires, you notice a direct, tangible improvement in your speed and bike-handling abilities. With stretching, it takes consistency and dedication to reap the performance benefits. Your goal has to be to get over the initial hump and make dynamic stretching a part of your daily routine. The exercises that follow have been precisely designed for that, as they are all cycling specific.

Dynamic Stretching Exercises

Although the core strength routines in this book are quite short, you still need to warm up your muscles properly with dynamic stretches before starting your core strength program. The dynamic stretches outlined here target the muscles that are traditionally the tightest on cyclists: hamstrings, low back, iliotibial (IT) band, chest, and shoulders. In addition to lengthening tight and inhibited muscles, these stretches will also help activate the lazy muscles of the glute complex and the low abs. By starting each core strength routine with a few dynamic stretches, you will increase your body's ability to perform the strengthening exercises correctly, which in turn will help you reach your core strength goals faster.

Stretches are often performed hurriedly and without intention. Don't fall into this common pattern of indifference. Remember that the point of dynamic stretching is to wake up the muscles and prepare them for work; if you are sleeping through the warm-up, you will lose the full benefit. Be mindful of the "muscles targeted" listed for each stretch, and focus on lengthening and engaging these areas. Clear your mind of other thoughts and concentrate on performing the exercises correctly and completely.

Also, when you are performing these stretches as your warm-up before the core routines in Chapters 6 through 8, be sure to follow the tempo that is assigned to each dynamic stretch in the core routine tables. Tempo is the suggested speed with which you perform the exercise; for a full explanation, see the section on tempo that begins on page 91 in the next chapter.

1 ▷ KNEELING QUAD STRETCH TO HAMSTRING STRETCH

GOAL > Increase muscle activation in the hips and legs; release chronic tightness in target muscle groups.

Come to a lunge position, with your left knee on the ground and your right foot planted in front of you Ⓐ. Your right leg should form a 90-degree angle at the knee joint. Maintain proper posture in your upper body by holding your ears over your shoulders, aligning your shoulders over your hips, and dropping your tailbone toward the ground. Shoulder blades should be pulled together slightly, and your chest should be open and slightly lifted.

Relax your right hand at your side and reach your left hand up to the ceiling, creating a long line from the left knee straight up through the left fingertips. As you continue to reach the left fingertips a few inches higher, tuck the tailbone again and gently push your hips forward until you feel a deep stretch in the front of the left leg.

Start the transition to the hamstring stretch by dropping your left hand down to your side. Slowly begin to sit back onto your left heel while beginning to straighten your right leg. Allow the toes of your right foot to come off the ground and point to the ceiling.

As you sit back, let both hands come down to the ground Ⓑ. If your hamstrings are tight, your right knee will remain bent; the goal is to eventually get the right leg as straight as possible.

Once you reach the end of your hamstring flexibility on the right leg, slowly rock forward into the lunge position again. Complete the number of repetitions designated in the core routine programs and then switch sides and repeat.

MUSCLES TARGETED

Quads, hamstrings, glutes, calves

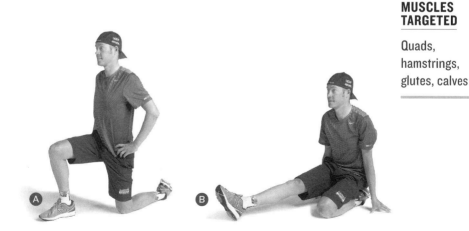

2 ▶ LOW-BACK STRETCH IN DOORWAY

GOAL > Increase range of motion in the low back; release chronic tightness in targeted muscle groups.

Hold on to a doorjamb (or a very sturdy pole of some sort) by placing your left hand on the inside of the doorjamb at chest height. Your palm should be facing away from your body. Now place your right hand 12 inches below your left. The rest of your body should be parallel to the door, with your feet hip distance apart.

Keeping your feet planted, gently begin to push your hips back as if you're trying to get your tailbone as far away from your hands as possible. Bend your knees while you are pushing your tailbone back so that you end up in a squat position Ⓐ.

From this position, begin to walk your hands up the doorjamb 2 inches at a time until you reach the top of your range (don't come out of your squat position) Ⓑ.

Slowly walk your hands down to the starting position and then continue to walk them as far down the doorjamb as possible, being sure to keep your squat position the entire time Ⓒ, Ⓓ.

Repeat this walking motion with the hands for the suggested number of repetitions, and then move to the other side of the doorjamb and repeat with the right hand above the left hand.

**MUSCLES
TARGETED**

Low back,
obliques

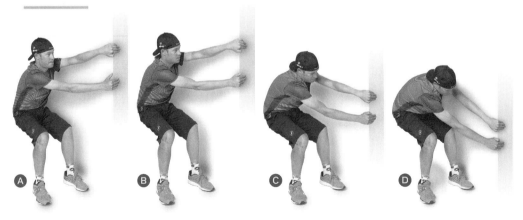

3 ▸ CHEST STRETCH AGAINST WALL

GOAL > Correct the "cycling slouch"; open up the chest cavity.

Stand with your body perpendicular to a wall so that the entire right side of your body is approximately 4 inches away from the wall. Without moving your lower body or twisting your torso toward the wall, reach your left arm straight behind you at shoulder height and rest your left palm on the wall. Now reach your right arm straight ahead of you at shoulder height and place your right palm on the wall. Both thumbs should be pointed toward the ceiling Ⓐ.

Gently remove your right hand from the wall and begin to swing it as far out to the right as you can, keeping your arm straight and at shoulder height Ⓑ.

As your chest and shoulders gain flexibility, you will be able to move your right hand farther and farther behind your body Ⓒ, so that eventually you won't be able to see your hand in your peripheral vision Ⓓ. When you've hit your reach limit, return your right hand to the wall in front of you.

Complete the suggested number of repetitions on this side and then turn around and repeat on the other side.

MUSCLES TARGETED

Shoulders, chest

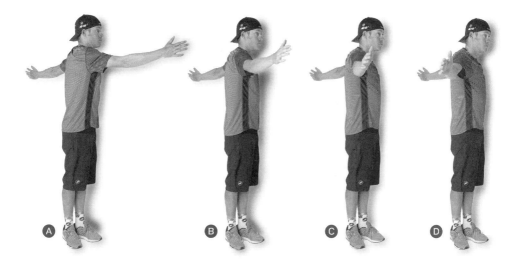

Ⓐ   Ⓑ   Ⓒ   Ⓓ

4 RAINBOW STRETCH IN DOORWAY

GOAL > Release chronic tightness in the IT band; increase lateral range of motion in the hips.

Stand in a doorway with the left side of your body approximately 6 inches away from the doorjamb. Cross your left foot over your right and place it flat on the ground, bending your knees slightly (A).

Place your left hand on the doorjamb at waist height. Slowly begin to reach your right hand up and over your head in a rainbow motion (B) and gently push your hips out to the right at the same time (C), (D). The goal is to form a letter "C" with your body and to touch the doorjamb above your head with your right hand (E). Return to starting position and repeat the suggested number of repetitions on this side.

Move to the other side of the doorway, cross your right foot over your left, and repeat by taking your left hand up and overhead.

MUSCLES TARGETED

Obliques, lats, shoulders, lateral hip muscles

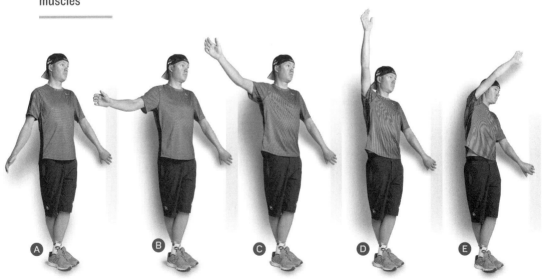

5 ▶ SUPINE FIGURE 4

GOAL > Release chronic tightness in the lumbo-pelvic-hip complex; increase muscle activation in the glutes.

Lie faceup on a mat or carpet with both legs extended out straight along the ground. Bend your right leg and place your right ankle on top of your left knee (be sure not to place it right on the kneecap, but rather above it) Ⓐ. Slowly bend your left leg and start to move it in toward your chest while you gently push your right knee farther out to the right.

When you are first starting, try reaching behind your left leg with your left hand and pulling in while your right hand gently pushes your right

knee away from your body Ⓑ. You should have the sensation of pulling with your left hand and pushing with your right.

Release your left leg back to the ground, but keep your right ankle on top of the left knee. Pull the left knee back in and repeat the push/pull with the hands.

Perform the suggested number of repetitions on this side, then switch.

MUSCLES TARGETED

Low back, glutes, lateral hip muscles

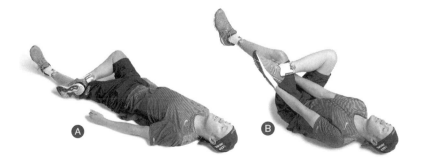

CHAPTER 5

Getting Started

You read the scientific rationale for developing a strong and efficient core in Part I, and now you're ready to put it all together. It may be tempting to just spin the core exercise wheel and see where you land, but taking an organized, progressive approach to your core routine will yield faster, more tangible results. The programs outlined in the following three chapters will show you how to approach your core strength training in a logical, safe, effective manner.

The programs have been divided into Levels I, II, and III. Within each level, there are five routines that focus on the following areas:

1. Injury Prevention/Rehab
2. Posture Correction
3. Stability and Bike Handling
4. Endurance
5. Tommy D's Optimum Performance Workout

Each routine begins with a 3-minute dynamic warm-up and is followed by 4 to 6 exercises. Most of the workouts take only 15 minutes to complete except for the Endurance Workout, which takes 25 minutes. No equipment is required, meaning that you have no excuse for skipping your core workout. Find a carpeted area or grab a yoga mat and get to work!

Deciding Which Level and Program Are Right for You

Okay, gearheads, this is the part where you check your ego at the door. Just because you can sustain a 15 percent incline for 30 minutes without blinking doesn't mean that you can rock a Level III core routine right out of the gate. If you jump into a core routine that is too advanced for your current strength level, you will be frustrated, embarrassed, and probably injured. Even the best cyclists in the world have to start with the basics when they are embarking on a core strengthening program. Same goes for you.

To accurately determine where to start, review the requirements for each level in Table 5.1. **You must meet at least two requirements to qualify for a level.**

Once you've established which level to start with, it's time to choose your workout. A suitable progression is to start with Workout 1 in Level I, II, or III and move through each workout in numerical order until you reach Workout 5 in that Level. The best progression of all would be to start with Workout 1, Level I at the

TABLE 5.1 CORE ROUTINE PLACEMENT TEST

LEVEL I	LEVEL II	LEVEL III
You have little to no experience with core strength training.	You have been doing core strength training regularly for at least 4 weeks.	You have been doing core strength training regularly for at least 8 weeks.
You can maintain a TT Position Hold (p. 120) for up to 20 seconds with good form.	You can maintain a TT Position Hold for 20–30 seconds with good form.	You can maintain a TT Position Hold for longer than 30 seconds with good form.
It is difficult for you to squeeze your shoulder blades together.	You can squeeze your shoulder blades together and hold for 5 seconds.	You can squeeze your shoulder blades together and hold for longer than 10 seconds.

> **TOMMY'S** TAKE Sometimes it's fun to get into the gym and play around with the equipment for my core routine, but most of the time I need something that I can do anywhere, anytime, especially when I'm on the road. That's one of the things I really appreciate about Allison's program designs: She always takes into account that I'm dragging my bike all over the world with me, so the last thing I need to do is take even more equipment along for the ride!

beginning of your off season and make it to Workout 5 (Tommy D's Optimum Performance Workout), Level III, at the same time you are reaching the height of your cycling training/racing. However, this progression may not be possible, or it may not be appropriate for your specific goals.

If you don't have any current injuries or concerns about possible overuse injuries, try to start with Workout 2 (Posture Correction) in whichever level you've reached. Resist the urge to skip Workout 2 and start with a "sexier" workout, unless you absolutely, without a doubt, already have perfect posture. If you aren't sure about your posture, refer back to page 65 for a guide to identifying your own postural distortions. Regardless of the type or amount of postural distortions you may be currently exhibiting, the routine outlined in Workout 2 (whether Level I, II, or III) will help to correct all of them.

In the rare instance that you have no postural distortions whatsoever, you are free to start with Workout 3, 4, or 5. Look at the "Goals" that are listed under each workout to decide which routine is in line with your own goals.

When to Move to the Next Level or Program

The amount of time spent in each level and on each workout program will vary from person to person, and will also be influenced by your goals at any particular point in time. However, a general rule of thumb is that you should spend at least 4 weeks on a workout before moving to a different one. You will know that it's time to move to a different workout when the exercises get easier, and when you feel yourself going into autopilot because the movements are so familiar.

If you have a particular area of concern (very poor posture, for example) then you can stay with the same workout number (in the case of posture, Workout 2) and simply move up through the different levels. Start with Workout 2 in Level I, follow this routine for a minimum of 4 weeks or until the exercises get easier, then move to Workout 2 in Level II.

The exercise variables (sets, reps, tempo, rest) have been laid out in a manner that becomes more challenging from one level to the next. With each level, the complexity of the exercises is increased, as is the total number of sets and reps. While the volume of work is increased, the amount of rest you are allowed is decreased; this trains the core musculature to simultaneously become stronger and have more endurance. After all, the ultimate goal of cycling is to be as strong as possible for as long as possible. These workouts will help facilitate that goal.

If you aren't focusing on one goal for an extended period of time, you will want to stay in the same level but switch workouts. For example, you may start with Workout 1 in Level II to address back pain; once that pain has decreased or disappeared, you can move on to another workout in Level II. It's very important to stay within the correct level even if you are switching workouts, since progressing to the next level too quickly can result in injury. Always refer to the Core Routine Placement Test (Table 5.1) on page 86 to decide if you're ready for the next level.

TOMMY'S TAKE One of the comforting things about being a pro athlete is that no matter how good you are at your sport, everyone you're competing against is going through the same amount of relative pain. I know that if I'm experiencing a 9 on a scale of I to IO, most of my competitors are as well. The same is true for you—regardless of your fitness level or cycling experience, your 9 still feels like a 9, so you and I are essentially both experiencing the same relative amount of discomfort. My point is this: Don't be afraid of trying something new (like these core workouts), because it's going to be challenging and frustrating. Every day that you can work on your fitness is a gift, so don't fight the pain—welcome it! Now get to work on your core strength and embrace the 9.

Working on Multiple Goals at Once

Are you confused about which workout to choose because you want to address posture, stability, and performance all at the same time? Good news: You can. The workout programs are designed to be multifaceted in their approach to core strength and fitness. For example, the design of Workout 1, Level I, focuses on preventing or decreasing aches and pains, but it simultaneously works on establishing strength throughout the entire core, which will then be put to use on the bike. You can almost think of the workouts as a gear cassette; you may spend most of your time in one cog, but that gear is flanked by other sprockets that you can shift to when necessary.

If none of the sample workouts seems to fit exactly what you're looking for, feel free to customize a workout on your own, or have a qualified trainer or strength coach put one together for you. When customizing your own workout, be sure to keep in mind the importance of the exercise variables and how these help determine the outcome of your workout. A detailed explanation of the workout variables, or terms, is in the following section. Read through this section carefully so you get a better idea of how exercise selection, number of reps, tempo, and rest period all need to be factored into a customized routine.

For example, if you know you have poor posture but you also want to work on optimum performance, you can try one of Tommy D's Optimum Performance Workouts and tack on some of the additional exercises that are included in the Posture Workout. It's essentially a matter of how much time and effort you are willing and able to put into meeting multiple goals at once.

Explanation of Terms Used in the Workout Programs

There are seven columns in each workout routine (see Table 5.2 for the routine headings). The descriptions for each appear in Table 5.2.

TABLE 5.2 SAMPLE WORKOUT ROUTINE HEADINGS

TYPE	EXERCISE	MUSCLES TARGETED	SETS	REPS	TEMPO	REST

Type: The first column tells you which part of the workout you're doing. These programs are fairly uncomplicated because there are only two types: Dynamic Warm-Up and Workout.

Exercise: The second column lists the particular exercise to be performed. The exercises themselves immediately follow the workouts, with written descriptions and pictures of Tommy D showing you how to do them.

Muscles targeted: This column lists the muscles and areas of the body most used with the particular exercise. Because the core musculature is so complex and interconnected, it is next to impossible to do an exercise that truly works only one muscle group at a time. Instead of listing every single agonist, synergist, and antagonist muscle involved, the primary muscle(s) being worked are listed so that you can balance your routine if you choose to perform only certain exercises; you can also refer to this column to select workouts that emphasize certain muscles.

Sets and reps: The fourth and fifth columns outline the total number of sets and repetitions that should be completed. A set is a group of repetitions, and a set should always be performed without rest. For example, in Workout 2 for Level I, you will perform 2 sets of 15 repetitions of Prone Snow Angels, with 30 seconds rest between each set. This means that you will complete 15 repetitions of Prone Snow Angels, rest 30 seconds, and then complete another 15 repetitions. Note that some exercises (TT Position Hold, for example) call for only 1 set, but you will be holding each of the repetitions in that set for a designated period of time and taking your rest period between each repetition. In this manner, you will complete a TT Position Hold for 5 seconds, rest 5 seconds, then hold for another 5 seconds, rest for 5 seconds, and so on.

Tempo: Tells you how fast each exercise should be performed. Tempo is a critical aspect of developing proper core strength, and it's often overlooked. If you perform an exercise too quickly, the proper muscles may not be recruited, and you could end up perpetuating a muscular imbalance or a postural distortion that you are trying to correct. A basic crunch is the perfect example; if you have ever heard someone bragging about how he does 500 crunches a day, you can bet those crunches are being pounded out at lightning speed with no awareness of form. Take that same person and ask him to do just 20 crunches at a speed of 3 seconds up and 3 seconds down, and he will be quivering by rep number 10. Why? Because he actually had to use his rectus abdominal muscles to lift his torso off the ground as opposed to throwing himself upward with momentum. Furthermore, a crunch performed too quickly is most likely being done by pushing the chin forward, which causes the muscles in the front of the neck to contract, which in turn pulls the head forward and perpetuates an exaggerated forward curvature in the cervical spine.

Most of the numbers in the Tempo column look like fractions—2/2 or 3/3—and these numbers represent how many seconds it should take to perform the concentric and eccentric contractions. A "concentric contraction" is the part of the movement that makes the muscle fiber shorter, which produces force. Think of picking up a backpack with your cycling gear inside. When you lift the bag off the ground, you grab the center handle or a strap and perform a bicep curl in order to bring the bag up toward your body. By flexing (concentric contraction) your biceps, you produced enough force to lift the bag.

When you set that bag back down on the floor, you are performing the eccentric part of a bicep curl. The term "eccentric" is not just used to describe your crazy Aunt Myrtle with the pet lizard; in strength training, eccentric (pronounced "E-sen-trik") refers to the lengthening of a muscle. An eccentric bicep contraction allows you to reduce force, or slow down force, as you set down your backpack.

Increasing your ability to dynamically reduce force will not only help optimize your core strength, it will also translate into more power on the bike. This can best be demonstrated by considering the role on the bike of the rectus abdominis muscle (the long, flat muscle that runs the length of your abdomen). There has been extensive discussion in this book about how cyclists always have tight, short rectus abdominis muscles owing to the number of hours spent on a bike in a hunched-over position. The concentric contraction of this muscle flexes the spine, thus pulling you into that hunched position—it's essentially an ab crunch. As important as this concentric role is, the eccentric role of the rectus abdominis is equally helpful for cyclists, mainly because it acts to decelerate spinal extension and spinal rotation. What this means for you is that when you stand up out of the saddle, or look over your shoulder in either direction, your body is able to do that without having your spine snap up or around too quickly, which could cause disc damage and pulled muscles, not to mention unwanted crashes.

The bottom line about tempo is this: Don't perform the exercises mindlessly and without any attention to how fast you're moving. If the exercise feels extremely easy and like something you could do all day long, you're probably moving too fast and letting momentum take over. Slow it down, breathe deeply, and count out the proper number of seconds for both the concentric and eccentric portions of the movement.

Rest: This column lists the suggested time to rest between reps. Note that there is no need to rest between dynamic warm-up exercises.

How to Incorporate the Core Workouts into Your Cycling Schedule

At the top of each workout you will find instructions for how many times per week you should complete the routine. The core strength routines in this book are slightly different from a whole-body strength routine, in that they don't involve additional weight and, therefore, don't require you to rest long between workouts. Also, because the muscles of the core are predominantly Type I endurance fibers, they can take more regular work without being at risk of injury. This means that you can do the core routines on consecutive days. Note, however, that it is advisable to take a rest day at least every third or fourth day.

TOMMY'S TAKE For me, the best way to keep up my core strength is to do the workouts in the morning, the day after a hard stage. Sometimes when I wake up the day after a hard race, I feel a little lethargic, achy, and mentally fuzzy. Once I have a little breakfast and coffee (lots of coffee) in me, doing my core routine after I digest is an effective way for me to get over the mental fuzziness and make a neuromuscular connection again.

The time of day that you do the core routine is your choice. If you know you will be physically exhausted at the end of the day, try to do the core routine in the morning so that your mind and body feel fresh. Remember that performing the exercises correctly and at the proper tempo are critical for achieving optimum results, so don't schedule your core routine at the point in the day when you know you're at your lowest energy level.

The core routines should be performed before a bike ride if at all possible. Many of the exercises are designed to improve muscle-firing patterns and to wake up important muscles that have been shut off. If you do a core routine right before you head out on a ride, those muscles will be alert, and you'll have all hands on deck for your cycling workout. You will quickly discover that a core routine before a bike ride is an effective warm-up that leads to improved performance.

CHAPTER 6

Level I Workouts and Exercises

There are several areas of concentration with the Level I workouts, but the two predominant goals are to establish motor neuron control in the core musculature and to activate muscles that have been shut off because of poor posture, injury, or chronic overuse. This may sound tedious and unexciting, but let's face it: You aren't reading this book to prepare for your swimsuit modeling session; you're reading this book to become a strong, powerful cyclist. As any great athlete will confirm, working on your strengths and ignoring your weaknesses is never an effective strategy for success. If you want to build a strong core, it will take diligence and commitment, and the Level I workouts represent the first step in that journey.

Workouts 1 and 2 place a big emphasis on activating the muscles of the kinetic chain that are traditionally weakest on a cyclist: transversus abdominals, low back, middle back, and glutes. The goal is to establish some awareness of these muscles and to work on holding a contraction for a period of 5 to 10 seconds. Because these muscles have probably been shut off for quite some time, it's important to start with 1 to 2 sets and to take adequate rest periods between sets so that your form doesn't suffer. One of the primary causes of overuse injuries is poor form, which increases dramatically as fatigue sets in. For this reason, more is not necessarily better when it comes to sets and reps in Workouts 1 and 2. Follow the parameters outlined, and you will set yourself up for success.

In Workout 3 we transition to a protocol that requires the core muscles to stabilize and engage during movement, which is exactly what those muscles should be doing when you're on the bike. Additionally, this workout starts to address the incredibly important concept of "intramuscular coordination." It sounds like a complicated term, but it simply means that you will be doing exercises that require different muscle groups to coordinate with each other and perform their respective functions at the same time. Think of it as a well-rehearsed choir of 20 voices; each voice is singing a different note, yet all of those notes come together to form a pleasing harmony.

Workout 4 is designed to challenge the endurance of the core musculature, hence the increased number of repetitions, which in turn increases the total workout time to 25 minutes. This is the longest workout in Level I, and for good reason. The abdominal muscles are composed primarily of Type I endurance fibers, which means they need to be worked primarily in an endurance fashion in order to see optimum results. In Workout 4, you will have the opportunity not only to increase your total time to fatigue, but also to address any lingering strength discrepancies between the right and left hemispheres of your body. All but one of the exercises in Level I, Workout 4, is performed unilaterally. This allows the muscles of the core to build strength independently and not to rely on the strength of the dominant side to do all the work.

TOMMY'S TAKE

I have to admit that my least favorite exercise is the TVA Activation. When I'm cycling, I feel confident in my strength and ability—I know I'm above average. But when I'm doing the TVA Activation, I feel really weak and below average, especially when compared to Allison . . . and the 90-year-olds in the gym rockin' out core routines like it's their job.

On the other hand, I really love doing the Low Back Stretch in Doorway. I feel it uses a natural movement that effectively stretches all the muscles that are ignored both on and off the bike. Plus, it allows me to get a great stretch without taxing my brain too much; I already get enough of that on the bike!

Workout 5 in Level I is a smorgasbord of exercises that help to establish optimum power, strength, and endurance. As with the endurance workout, you will still be performing 3 sets of each exercise, but now the reps have been taken down slightly (from 15 to 12) and the complexity of the exercises has been increased. The emphasis is still on addressing the chronically weak and underused muscles of the posterior, while also working the entire core musculature.

LEVEL I, WORKOUT 1 | INJURY PREVENTION/REHAB WORKOUT

GOAL > To decrease pain, increase neuromuscular efficiency, and address long-standing muscular imbalances that cause injury.

TYPE	EXERCISE	MUSCLES TARGETED	SETS	REPS	TEMPO	REST
DYNAMIC WARM-UP	Low-Back Stretch in Doorway (p. 80)	Low back, obliques	1	3 up and down each side	3/3	None
	Rainbow Stretch in Doorway (p. 82)	Obliques, lats, shoulders, lateral hip muscles	1	10 each side	3/3	None
	Supine Figure 4 (p. 83)	Low back, glutes, lateral hip muscles	1	10 each leg	2/2	None
WORKOUT	Opposite Arm/ Leg Reach (p. 106)	Low back, glute major	2	10 each side	2/2	30 seconds
	Hip Bridge with Heel Slides (p. 109)	Low back, hamstrings, glutes	2	10 each leg	2/2	30 seconds
	TVA Activation (p. 112)	Transversus abdominis (TVA)	1	5	Hold 5 seconds	5 seconds between each rep
	Tailbone Tucks (p. 113)	Transversus abdominis (TVA)	1	5	Hold 5 seconds	5 seconds between each rep

FREQUENCY > 3–5 times per week   **TOTAL WORKOUT TIME >** 12 minutes

LEVEL I, WORKOUT 2	POSTURE-CORRECTION WORKOUT

GOAL > To correct muscular tightness and weakness, improve joint mobility, and establish optimum positioning of the spinal column.

TYPE	EXERCISE	MUSCLES TARGETED	SETS	REPS	TEMPO	REST
DYNAMIC WARM-UP	Kneeling Quad to Hamstring Stretch (p. 79)	Quads, hamstrings, glutes, calves	I	IO each leg	3/3	None
	Chest Stretch Against Wall (p. 81)	Shoulders, chest	I	IO each arm	3/3	None
	Rainbow Stretch in Doorway (p. 82)	Obliques, lats, shoulders, lateral hip muscles	I	IO each side	3/3	None
WORKOUT	Prone Snow Angels (p. 108)	Low back, mid back, hip abductors	2	I5	2/2	30 seconds
	Shoulder Blade Squeeze (p. 110)	Mid back	I	IO	Hold 5 seconds	5 seconds between each rep
	Wall Squat with Pelvic Tucks (p. 114)	Transversus abdominis (TVA)	I	IO	Hold 5 seconds	5 seconds between each rep
	Pac-Mans (p. 117)	Lateral hip muscles	2	I5 each leg	3/3	30 seconds
	Chair Squats (p. 119)	Entire core musculature	2	I5	2/2	30 seconds

FREQUENCY > 3–5 times per week   **TOTAL WORKOUT TIME >** I5 minutes

LEVEL I, WORKOUT 3 > STABILITY AND BIKE-HANDLING WORKOUT

GOAL > To improve static and dynamic stabilization of the entire core musculature, increase muscle-firing efficiency, and improve intramuscular coordination.

TYPE	EXERCISE	MUSCLES TARGETED	SETS	REPS	TEMPO	REST
DYNAMIC WARM-UP	Low-Back Stretch in Doorway (p. 80)	Low back, obliques	1	10 each side	3/3	None
	Chest Stretch Against Wall (p. 81)	Shoulders, chest	1	10 each arm	3/3	None
	Rainbow Stretch in Doorway (p. 82)	Obliques, lats, shoulders, lateral hip muscles	1	10 each side	3/3	None
WORKOUT	Supermans (p. 107)	Low back, glute major	2	12	2/2	30 seconds
	Mountain Climbers (p. 111)	Transversus abdominis (TVA), hip flexors, quads	2	12 each leg	2/2	30 seconds
	Side Planks (p. 115)	Obliques	2	12 each side	2/2	30 seconds
	Audrey Two (p. 118)	Lateral hip muscles	2	12 each leg	2/2	30 seconds
	TT Position Hold (p. 120)	Entire core musculature	2	1	Hold for 20–30 seconds	30 seconds

FREQUENCY > 2–3 times per week   **TOTAL WORKOUT TIME** > 17 minutes

LEVEL I, WORKOUT 4	ENDURANCE WORKOUT

GOAL > To improve muscular endurance and efficiency of the core and increase time to exhaustion.

TYPE	EXERCISE	MUSCLES TARGETED	SETS	REPS	TEMPO	REST
DYNAMIC WARM-UP	Kneeling Quad to Hamstring Stretch (p. 79)	Quads, hamstrings, glutes, calves	1	10 each leg	3/3	None
	Chest Stretch Against Wall (p. 81)	Shoulders, chest	1	10 each arm	3/3	None
	Rainbow Stretch in Doorway (p. 82)	Obliques, lats, shoulders, lateral hip muscles	1	10 each side	3/3	None
WORKOUT	Hip Bridge with Heel Slides (p. 109)	Low back, hamstrings, glutes	2	15 each leg	2/2	30 seconds
	Mountain Climbers (p. 111)	Transversus abdominis (TVA), hip flexors, quads	2	15 each leg	2/2	30 seconds
	Supine Knee Drops (p. 116)	Obliques, low back	2	15 each side	2/2	30 seconds
	Pac-Mans (p. 117)	Lateral hip muscles	2	15 each leg	2/2	30 seconds
	TT Position Hold (p. 120)	Entire core musculature	2	1	Hold 30–40 seconds	30 seconds

FREQUENCY > 2–3 times per week   **TOTAL WORKOUT TIME** > 25 minutes

LEVEL I, WORKOUT 5 > TOMMY D'S OPTIMUM PERFORMANCE WORKOUT

GOAL > To develop optimum core strength, increase power production, improve muscular endurance, and be able to keep up with Tom while he climbs Alpe d'Huez.

TYPE	EXERCISE	MUSCLES TARGETED	SETS	REPS	TEMPO	REST
DYNAMIC WARM-UP	Low-Back Stretch in Doorway (p. 80)	Low back, obliques	1	3 each side	3/3	None
	Rainbow Stretch in Doorway (p. 82)	Obliques, lats, shoulders, lateral hip muscles	1	10 each side	3/3	None
	Supine Figure 4 (p. 83)	Low back, glutes, lateral hip muscles	1	10 each leg	3/3	None
WORKOUT	Prone Snow Angels (p. 108)	Low back, mid back, hip abductors	2	12	2/2	30 seconds
	Hip Bridge with Heel Slides (p. 109)	Low back, hamstrings, glutes	2	12 each leg	2/2	30 seconds
	Mountain Climbers (p. 111)	Transversus abdominis (TVA), hip flexors, quads	2	12 each leg	2/2	30 seconds
	Side Planks (p. 115)	Obliques	2	12 each side	2/2	30 seconds
	Chair Squats (p. 119)	Entire core musculature	2	12	2/2	30 seconds

FREQUENCY > 3–4 times per week   **TOTAL WORKOUT TIME** > 20 minutes

LEVEL I EXERCISE EXPLANATIONS

The Level I exercises have been carefully selected to provide you with an effective, safe, scientifically based place in which to begin building core strength. If you are starting with Level I, you probably haven't been doing core training with much frequency (maybe not at all), so the emphasis will be on lengthening the tight and inhibited muscles on the front side of the body while simultaneously building strength and muscular integrity on the back of the body.

Throw away your old core routines that were based on traditional crunches and sit-ups, and step into a more holistic, functional approach to core training. You will notice that the Level I exercises emphasize the low back, glutes, deep abdominals, low abs, and obliques, all of which are typically ignored in a traditional core strength program. Crunch-type movements usually require you to lie on your back and lift your upper body by curling your spine toward your knees. This is exactly the type of movement you want to avoid, because it only perpetuates that hunched-over position you are already holding for hours on end while you ride. Instead, the goal of the Level I exercises is to reverse all those postural distortions, poor muscle-firing patterns, and injuries that result from having an overactive rectus abdominis.

Several of the exercises in Level I ask you to hold a certain position for several seconds, which helps to establish a mind-muscle connection with muscles that have probably been shut off for quite some time. Don't go into Level I thinking it will be easy—you will be challenged and sore just like the first time you tackled a big ride!

LEVEL I EXERCISES

EXERCISE NUMBER		EXERCISE NAME	MUSCLES TARGETED
1		Opposite Arm/Leg Reach	Low back, glute major
2		Supermans	Low back, glute major
3		Prone Snow Angels	Low back, middle back, hip abductors
4		Hip Bridge with Heel Slides	Low back, glutes, hamstrings
5		Shoulder Blade Squeeze	Middle back
6		Mountain Climbers	Transversus abdominis (TVA), hip flexors, quads
7		Transverse Abdominis (TVA) Activation	Transversus abdominis (TVA)
8		Tailbone Tucks	Transversus abdominis (TVA)

EXERCISE NUMBER		EXERCISE NAME	MUSCLES TARGETED
9		Wall Squat with Pelvic Tucks	Transversus abdominis (TVA)
10		Side Planks	Obliques
11		Supine Knee Drops	Obliques, low back
12		Pac Mans	Lateral hip muscles
13		Audrey Two	Lateral hip muscles
14		Chair Squats	Entire core musculature
15		TT Position Hold	Entire core musculature

1 ▶ OPPOSITE ARM/LEG REACH

GOAL > Improve intramuscular coordination between the core and the extremities; teach the core to use the glute major for hip extension.

Start in a quadruped position (on hands and knees), making sure that hands are directly below the shoulders and knees are directly below the hips Ⓐ. Keep the back of your neck long; do not look up or let your chin drop toward the ground. Activate the abdominal muscles by gently pulling your belly button up, being careful not to round your upper back at the same time.

Keep your hips and shoulders parallel to the ground and lift your right foot and left hand at the same time Ⓑ. Extend the fingertips forward and toes backward as far as possible. Squeeze your right glute. Hold this extension for 5 seconds and then bring your hand and foot down to the mat at the same time. Repeat on the other side Ⓒ, and continue alternating until you have completed the designated number of repetitions.

MUSCLES TARGETED

Low back, glute major

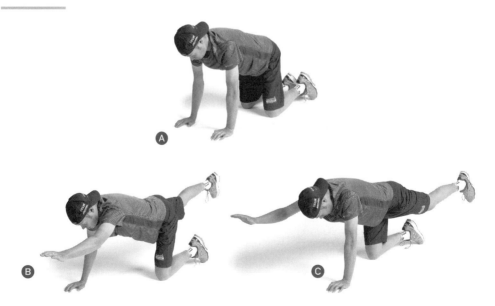

2 ▶ SUPERMANS

GOAL > Increase strength and range of motion in the low back; teach glutes and hamstrings to fire during hip extension.

Begin by lying facedown on the ground with arms extended above your head Ⓐ. Put space between your ears and your shoulders by dropping your shoulder blades down toward your waist.

Gently squeeze your glutes and slowly begin to raise your feet and hands off the ground Ⓑ. Do not lift more than 6 inches. Think about

pulling the top of your head and your tailbone in opposite directions. Hold this position at the top for 5 seconds and gently release.

Refresh your starting position each time by dropping the shoulder blades down the back before you lift. Repeat until you have completed the designated number of repetitions.

MUSCLES TARGETED

Low back, glute major

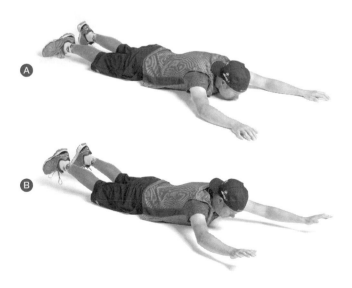

3 PRONE SNOW ANGELS

GOAL > Increase strength and range of motion in the low back; teach stabilization in the thoracic and cervical spine when the arms are moving.

The term "prone" means face down, which is the position of the body for this exercise. Start with the arms extended along your sides with palms down A. Keep the back of your neck long and your shoulder blades dropped down toward your waist.

Gently squeeze your glutes and slowly begin to raise your feet, chest, and hands off the ground B. Do not lift more than 6 inches. Create a "snow angel" by sweeping your arms overhead and separating your feet C. Without bending your arms, try to bring your hands all the way together above your head D. Return to starting position and allow your feet, chest, and hands to relax down to the ground E. Repeat until you have completed the designated number of repetitions.

If your shoulders and chest muscles are tight, you will not be able to touch your hands together at first. It's better to keep your arms straight and have your hands slightly separated above your head than to bend your arms and touch your hands.

MUSCLES TARGETED

Low back,
middle back,
hip abductors

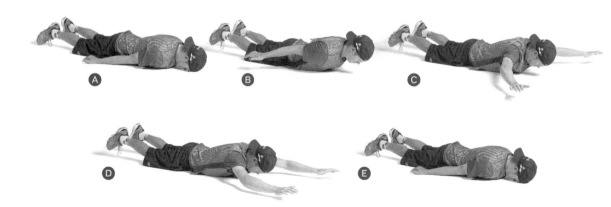

4 HIP BRIDGE WITH HEEL SLIDES

GOAL > Release chronic tightness on the front side of the body; teach the glutes and hamstrings to fire during hip extension.

Start on your back with your knees bent and feet on the ground approximately 6 to 8 inches from your glutes. Your arms should be relaxed on the ground at your sides Ⓐ.

Squeeze your glutes, tuck your tailbone, and lift your hips off the ground Ⓑ. Keeping your hips high, slide your right foot away from your

body until your leg is completely straight Ⓒ, then bring it back in.

Repeat this sliding motion with the left foot, keeping your hips stable the entire time Ⓓ.

Alternate back and forth between your feet until you have completed the designated number of repetitions.

MUSCLES TARGETED

Low back, glutes, hamstrings

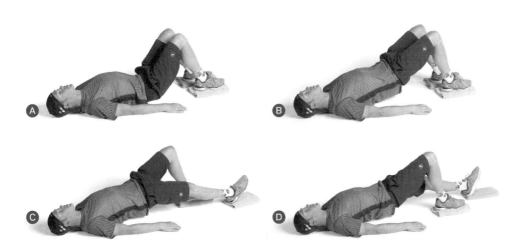

5 ▷ SHOULDER BLADE SQUEEZE

GOAL > Combat the cycling slouch; open up the chest cavity to facilitate better breathing.

Start on your hands and knees with your knees below your hips. Place your hands directly below your shoulders, as if you were going to do a push-up Ⓐ.

Keeping your arms straight, drop your shoulder blades down toward your waist and then squeeze them together Ⓑ. Don't let your low back sway or your chin push forward.

Hold the shoulder blade squeeze for 5 seconds and release. Repeat until you have completed the designated number of repetitions.

MUSCLES TARGETED

Middle back (specifically rhomboids)

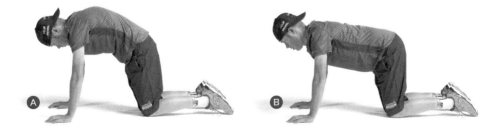

6 ⟩ MOUNTAIN CLIMBERS

GOAL > Teach the core muscles (specifically the TVA) to stabilize the pelvis while the legs are in motion.

Start in a push-up position with a small towel under each foot Ⓐ (if you are on a carpeted floor, place a small piece of cardboard under each foot). Avoid rounding in the upper back by squeezing your shoulder blades together, and do not push your chin forward. Lengthen through the spine and activate the TVA by pulling the lower abdominal area up toward the spine.

Without rocking or swaying your hips, slowly slide your right knee in toward your chest Ⓑ and slowly push back out. Wait until the right leg is back in starting position before you pull in the left knee Ⓒ. Keep a close eye on your upper and lower back positioning throughout the exercise, and don't forget to keep the hips steady. Continue switching legs until you have completed the designated number of repetitions.

MUSCLES TARGETED

Transversus abdominis, hip flexors, quads

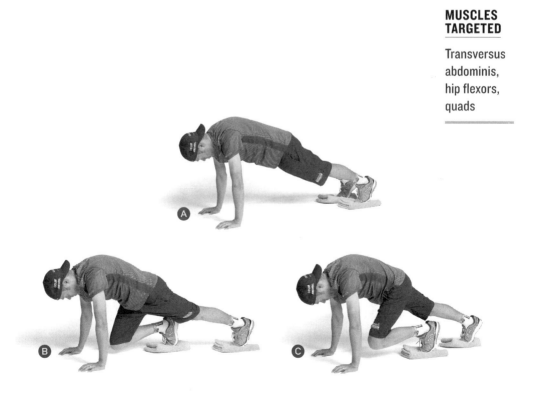

7 TRANSVERSUS ABDOMINIS (TVA) ACTIVATION

GOAL > Improve activation of the deep abdominal muscles (TVA); decrease chronic pain in the low back.

Start on your back with your knees bent and feet on the ground approximately 6 to 8 inches from your glutes (A). It is very important to keep your upper body totally relaxed during this exercise. Keep your head on the ground and keep your hands relaxed by your sides.

Gently begin to hollow out the area below your belly button by dropping your lower abs toward the ground (B). Do not forcefully pull in your abs, but rather think of creating a bowl between your belly button and your pubic bone. Concentrate on the area below the belly button and try to keep your upper abs relaxed.

Hold this for the designated amount of time and then release before moving to additional repetitions.

MUSCLES TARGETED

Transversus abdominis

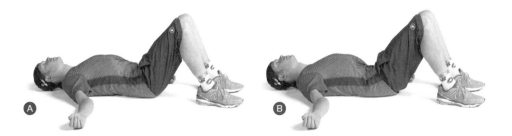

8 › TAILBONE TUCKS

GOAL > Isolate the TVA muscle and teach it to fire on command.

Start in a quadruped position (on hands and knees), making sure that your hands are directly below your shoulders and your knees are directly below your hips Ⓐ. Keep the back of your neck long; do not look up or let your chin drop toward the ground.

Without moving your rib cage, shoulders, neck, or head, gently drop your tailbone toward the ground while simultaneously pulling your belly button toward the spine Ⓑ. Hold this tucked position for the designated amount of time, then release.

MUSCLES TARGETED

Transversus abdominis

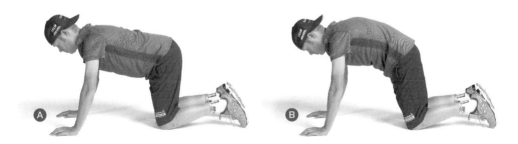

9 | WALL SQUAT WITH PELVIC TUCKS

GOAL > Teach the lower abdominal muscles (TVA) to fire on command when the leg muscles are engaged.

Start in a squat position against the wall (A). The goal is to reach a 90-degree angle at the knees, but if this position makes your knees hurt, you can slide up the wall a bit. The back of your head, shoulder blades, middle back, and glutes should all be touching the wall (B). There should be a slight curvature in the lower back that allows one hand to slide in and out, but no more than that.

Keeping all points of contact with the wall, slowly drop your tailbone toward the ground and pull in your lower abdominal area until that slight curvature in the low back disappears and you feel the low back touch the wall (C).

Hold this tuck for the designated amount of time, then release.

MUSCLES TARGETED

Transversus
abdominis

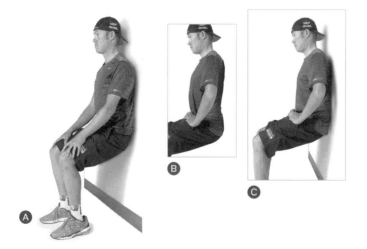

10 SIDE PLANKS

GOAL > Improve muscular activation of the internal obliques, which will help with bike stabilization while climbing out of the saddle.

Start on your right side with your right forearm on the ground, keeping your right elbow directly below your right shoulder Ⓐ. Keep your left leg straight and bend the right leg to a 90-degree angle Ⓑ. Create a straight line from your left shoulder all the way down to your left ankle. Check to make sure your hips are pushed forward, tailbone is tucked, and ears are directly above your shoulders.

Keeping your left hand on the ground in front of your chest for stability, push down through the right forearm and lift your hips off the ground Ⓒ. The right knee remains on the ground throughout this exercise to provide support for the low back. Lift the left hip up and down for the designated number of repetitions and then switch sides.

MUSCLES TARGETED

Obliques

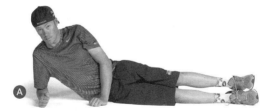

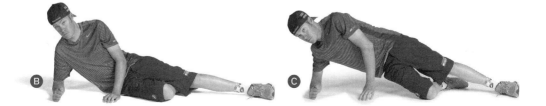

11 > SUPINE KNEE DROPS

GOAL > Release chronic tightness in the lower back and outer hips while simultaneously using the obliques to control movement.

Start in a supine position (lying on the ground, faceup) with the feet off the ground and legs forming a 90-degree angle at the hips and knees Ⓐ. Arms should extend out from the body in a "T" position.

Keeping your upper body relaxed, drop your knees as far to the left as possible without letting your right arm and shoulder blade come off the ground Ⓑ, Ⓒ. Return your legs to center and drop to the right Ⓓ, Ⓔ. Concentrate on trying to use your abdominal muscles to lift your legs off the ground.

Continue alternating side to side.

MUSCLES TARGETED

Obliques, low back

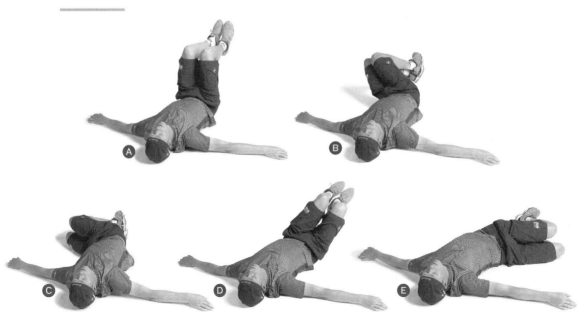

12 · PAC-MANS

GOAL > Increase strength and muscle activation in the chronically tight muscles of the outer hip.

This exercise got its name from the way Pac-Man eats up his competition. Start on your left side with the back of your body against a wall (A). Your head should be completely relaxed, either by laying it on your extended left arm or supporting it with your left hand. Points of contact with the wall should be heels, glutes, shoulder blades, and back of the head.

Place your right hand on your right hip and slowly begin to slide your right leg up the wall (this is abduction) . The goal is to use the muscles of the outer hip to lift the leg instead of lifting the entire pelvis. If you feel the hip bone on your right side moving upward toward your chest, you are lifting your pelvis. Complete the designated number of repetitions on this side, then switch.

MUSCLES TARGETED

Lateral hip muscles

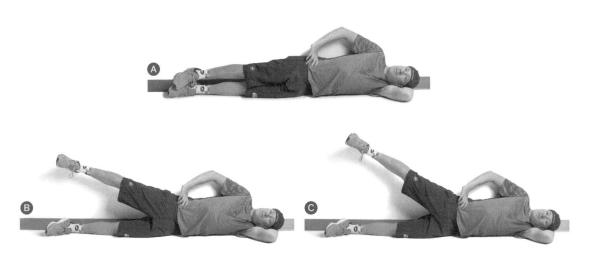

13 AUDREY TWO

GOAL > Teach the glute medius and TFL to fire while keeping the pelvis stable.

The Audrey Two is named after the hungry Venus fly trap featured in the movie *Little Shop of Horrors*. Think of your feet as the hinge at the back of Audrey Two's mouth and your knees as the part that eats up anything in its path. Start on your left side with the back of your body against a wall Ⓐ. Your head should be completely relaxed, either by laying it on your extended left arm or supporting it with your left hand. Bend both knees and place the bottoms of your feet against the wall. Points of contact

with the wall should be soles of the feet, glutes, shoulder blades, and back of the head.

Place your right hand on your right hip and slowly begin to open your right knee up toward the wall Ⓑ. Keep the ankles and feet pressed together the entire time, thus creating a "clam-opening" effect Ⓒ. Complete the designated number of repetitions on this side, then switch.

MUSCLES TARGETED

Lateral hip muscles

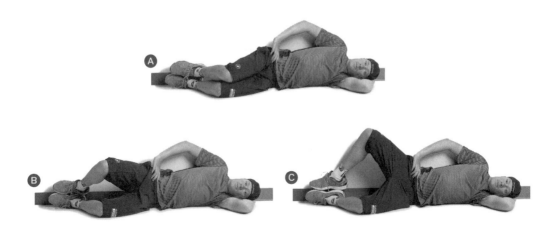

14 CHAIR SQUATS

GOAL > Teach the glutes and hamstrings to fire; reduce workload placed on the quadriceps.

A squat is one of the most common movements performed by humans. On a given day, you will do some variation of a squat movement approximately 50 to 100 times. Sound like a lot? Consider how many times you get in and out of a car, go to the bathroom, sit down on a chair, or bend down to pick up an object—all of these movements are variations on a squat. Because we perform squats so frequently, it is imperative that we are doing so with correct form in order to avoid putting undue stress on the knees and hips.

A safe and effective way to learn proper squat form is to use a chair as a safety net. Choose a chair with a seat that hits you approximately at knee height.

Stand in front of the chair with your feet hip distance apart, chest lifted, tailbone slightly

tucked, and hands on your hips Ⓐ. Pick your toes up inside your shoes and transfer all your weight into your heels. Push your hips back as far as possible before you start lowering down into the chair Ⓑ. Be sure that your knees don't come past your toes and your chest does not drop or cave in Ⓒ.

The goal is to eventually come all the way down and touch the chair Ⓓ, but when you first start you may only be able to lower down 12 inches or so before your form starts to waver.

Return to your standing position by driving weight down into your heels and lifting your chest first. Finish off the movement by squeezing your glutes as you reach starting position. Repeat until you have completed the designated number of repetitions.

MUSCLES TARGETED

Entire core musculature

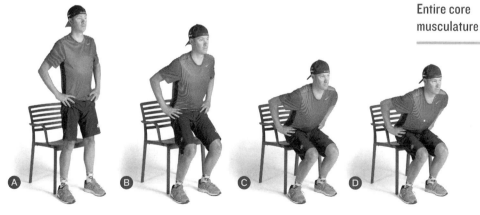

15 ❯ TT (TIME TRIAL) POSITION HOLD

GOAL > Engage all the muscles of the core equally; improve intramuscular coordination between the upper back, lower back, and lower abs.

You may know this exercise as a plank hold, but for cyclists, this position is most useful during a time trial or a fast descent. If you need to work on being more aerodynamic, this is your exercise.

The TT Hold is performed on your forearms and toes, and there is no movement, which makes it an isometric exercise. Your elbows should be directly beneath your shoulders, and your feet should be 8 to 10 inches apart Ⓐ. Keep the back of your neck long and look down at the floor.

Work to bring your shoulder blades onto your back by squeezing them together slightly; your upper back should not be rounded. Your lower back should not be excessively rounded either, nor should you adopt a swayback position. Hold this position for the designated amount of time, and remember to breathe!

MUSCLES TARGETED

Entire core musculature

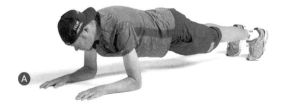

CHAPTER 7

Level II Workouts and Exercises

The Level II workouts are, as you would expect, more challenging than the Level I workouts in the previous chapter. Before you take on Level II, be sure to take the Placement Test on page 86 to confirm that you're ready for them.

Workout 1 in Level II is similar to its counterpart in Level I, in that the emphasis is still placed on correcting muscular imbalances and increasing neuromuscular efficiency. The main difference you will see in Level II is that you will be performing 2 sets of each exercise right out of the gate; if the Placement Test revealed you're ready for Level II, then you already have the muscular endurance necessary to perform 2 sets with good form. An additional change from Level I is that your injury-prevention exercises now require you to move instead of holding a contraction for 5 to 10 seconds.

Workout 2 in Level II is a bit more aggressive than Workout 2 in Level I, in that the exercises start to work into the shoulder girdle (Prone Snow Angel with Shoulder Press) as well as requiring the lateral hip muscles to fire from a standing position as opposed to lying on the ground. The exercise you might find to be a surprising challenge is the Shoulder Blade Squeeze from Push-up Position. Not only are you asked to perform the exercise from your toes instead of your knees, as in Level I, but the number of repetitions has also been increased.

Workout 3 is probably the most mentally demanding of all the Level II workouts. There are 6 exercises, all of which require varying levels of intramuscular coordination as well as balance and stability. Because these exercises are so physically and mentally demanding, you will only do 2 sets of each, with the exception of the 2 exercises that specifically work on balance and stability. Be sure to take your full 30 seconds of rest between each set, and feel free to increase that rest period if you sense your form is failing.

The Level II Endurance workout kicks it up a notch as well. Because one of the primary concerns with establishing endurance is to improve your time to fatigue, your rest periods in Level II will be cut from 30 to 20 seconds. The true mark of endurance is to be able to work hard and then recover quickly, and, with only 20 seconds to rest between sets, you will certainly be testing both your physical and mental stamina. Even if you can perform the workout with less rest between sets, keep in mind that blowing through exercises at lightning speed usually comes at the expense of proper form, which can lead to injury. Commit to spending 25 minutes with this workout, and know that your return on that investment will be well worth it.

And finally, there's Tommy D's Optimum Performance Workout for Level II. Now is when you're ready to start moving your body with a little quicker speed, but still maintain motor control and good form; many of the exercises have been taken from a 2/2 tempo to a 1/1 tempo. Don't let this quicker tempo encourage sloppiness. Instead, pull back on the reins and maintain focus on your form, your tempo, and using all of those new muscle-firing patterns you have created.

TOMMY'S TAKE

By the end of racing season, I have usually built up several nagging pains due to postural distortions. Neck, back, chest— if it's connected to my spine, it hurts! One of the areas that constantly seems to need adjustment from the team chiropractor is my thoracic area (middle back), which is why Allison always has me do the Shoulder Blade Squeeze exercise for the first month of my off-season. It's nice to reset my posture and get rid of all the damage that has been done during racing season.

LEVEL II, WORKOUT 1 >	INJURY PREVENTION/REHAB WORKOUT

GOAL > To decrease pain, increase neuromuscular efficiency, and address long-standing muscular imbalances that cause injury.

TYPE	EXERCISE	MUSCLES TARGETED	SETS	REPS	TEMPO	REST
DYNAMIC WARM-UP	Low-Back Stretch in Doorway (p. 80)	Low back, obliques	1	3 up and down each side	3/3	None
	Rainbow Stretch in Doorway (p. 82)	Obliques, lats, shoulders, lateral hip muscles	1	10 each side	3/3	None
	Supine Figure 4 (p. 83)	Low back, glutes, lateral hip muscles	1	10 each leg	2/2	None
WORKOUT	Opposite Arm/ Leg Reach from Plank Position (p. 131)	Low back, glute major	2	10 each side	2/2	30 seconds
	Walking Hip Bridge (p. 134)	Low back, hamstrings, glutes	2	10 each leg	2/2	30 seconds
	Tim-berrr! (p. 136)	Transversus abdominis (TVA)	2	10 each leg	2/2	30 seconds
	Reverse Crunch (p. 137)	Transversus abdominis (TVA)	2	15	2/2	30 seconds

FREQUENCY > 3–5 times per week   **TOTAL WORKOUT TIME** > 17 minutes

LEVEL II, WORKOUT 2 POSTURE-CORRECTION WORKOUT

GOAL > To correct muscular tightness and weakness, improve joint mobility, and establish optimum positioning of the spinal column.

TYPE	EXERCISE	MUSCLES TARGETED	SETS	REPS	TEMPO	REST
DYNAMIC WARM-UP	Kneeling Quad to Hamstring Stretch (p. 79)	Quads, hamstrings, glutes, calves	1	10 each leg	3/3	None
	Chest Stretch Against Wall (p. 81)	Shoulders, chest	1	10 each arm	3/3	None
	Rainbow Stretch in Doorway (p. 82)	Obliques, lats, shoulders, lateral hip muscles	1	10 each side	3/3	None
WORKOUT	Prone Snow Angels with Shoulder Press (p. 133)	Low back, mid back, upper back, shoulders, lateral hip muscles	2	10	2/2 for Angel, 1/1 for Press	30 seconds
	Shoulder Blade Squeeze from Push-up Position (p. 135)	Mid back	1	15	Hold 5 seconds	5 seconds between each rep
	Tim-berrr! (p. 136)	Transversus abdominis (TVA)	2	10 each leg	2/2	30 seconds
	Crossover Squats (p. 140)	Glutes, hamstrings, quads, lateral hip muscles	2	10 each leg	1/1	30 seconds
	TT Position Acceleration (p. 143)	Entire core musculature	2	10 each leg	1/1	30 seconds

FREQUENCY > 3–5 times per week   **TOTAL WORKOUT TIME** > 17 minutes

LEVEL II, WORKOUT 3	STABILITY AND BIKE-HANDLING WORKOUT

GOAL > To improve static and dynamic stabilization of the entire core musculature, increase muscle-firing efficiency, and improve intramuscular coordination.

TYPE	EXERCISE	MUSCLES TARGETED	SETS	REPS	TEMPO	REST
DYNAMIC WARM-UP	Low-Back Stretch in Doorway (p. 80)	Low back, obliques	1	10 each side	3/3	None
	Chest Stretch Against Wall (p. 81)	Shoulders, chest	1	10 each arm	3/3	None
	Rainbow Stretch in Doorway (p. 82)	Obliques, lats, shoulders, lateral hip muscles	1	10 each side	3/3	None
WORKOUT	Supermans with Heel Touches (p. 132)	Low back, glute major, hamstrings	2	10 each side	2/2	30 seconds
	Side Plank (p. 139)	Obliques	2	10 each side	2/2	30 seconds
	Crossover Squats (p. 140)	Glutes, hamstrings, quads, lateral hip muscles	2	10 each leg	1/1	30 seconds
	Grab the Water Bottle (p. 141)	Transversus abdominis (TVA), shoulder complex, spinal stabilizers	2	10 each side	2/2	30 seconds
	The Wall (p. 142)	Transversus abdominis (TVA), shoulder complex, spinal stabilizers	2	10 each side	2/2	30 seconds

FREQUENCY > 2–3 times per week   **TOTAL WORKOUT TIME** > 19 minutes

LEVEL II, WORKOUT 4	ENDURANCE WORKOUT

GOAL > To improve muscular endurance and efficiency of the core and increase time to exhaustion.

TYPE	EXERCISE	MUSCLES TARGETED	SETS	REPS	TEMPO	REST
DYNAMIC WARM-UP	Kneeling Quad to Hamstring Stretch (p. 79)	Quads, hamstrings, glutes, calves	1	10 each leg	3/3	None
	Chest Stretch Against Wall (p. 81)	Shoulders, chest	1	10 each arm	3/3	None
	Rainbow Stretch in Doorway (p. 82)	Obliques, lats, shoulders, lateral hip muscles	1	10 each side	3/3	None
WORKOUT	Walking Hip Bridge (p. 134)	Low back, hamstrings, glutes	2	15 each leg	2/2	20 seconds
	Reverse Crunch (p. 137)	Transversus abdominis (TVA)	2	15	2/2	20 seconds
	Seated Boat Row (p. 138)	Obliques	2	1 each side	Hold 15 seconds	20 seconds
	TT Position Acceleration (p. 143)	Entire core musculature	2	15 each leg	1/1	20 seconds
	Overhead Squats (p. 144)	Glute medius, lateral hips	2	15	2/2	20 seconds

FREQUENCY > 2–3 times per week   **TOTAL WORKOUT TIME** > 25 minutes

| LEVEL II, WORKOUT 5 | TOMMY D'S OPTIMUM PERFORMANCE WORKOUT |

GOAL > To develop optimum core strength, increase power production, improve muscular endurance, and be able to keep up with Tom while he climbs Alpe d'Huez.

TYPE	EXERCISE	MUSCLES TARGETED	SETS	REPS	TEMPO	REST
DYNAMIC WARM-UP	Low-Back Stretch in Doorway (p. 80)	Low back, obliques	1	3 each side	3/3	None
	Rainbow Stretch in Doorway (p. 82)	Obliques, lats, shoulders, lateral hip muscles	1	10 each side	3/3	None
	Supine Figure 4 (p. 83)	Low back, glutes, lateral hip muscles	1	10 each leg	3/3	None
WORKOUT	Prone Snow Angels with Shoulder Press (p. 133)	Low back, mid back, upper back, shoulders, lateral hip muscles	2	12	2/2 for Angel, 1/1 for Press	30 seconds
	Reverse Crunch (p. 137)	Transversus abdominis (TVA)	2	12	2/2	30 seconds
	Grab the Water Bottle (p. 141)	Transversus abdominis (TVA), shoulder complex, spinal stabilizers	2	12 each side	1/1	30 seconds
	Seated Boat Row (p. 138)	Obliques	2	1 each side	Hold 15 seconds each side	30 seconds
	Crossover Squats (p. 140)	Glute medius	2	12 each side	1/1	30 seconds
	TT Final Sprint (p. 145)	Entire core musculature	2	12 each arm	1/1	30 seconds

FREQUENCY > 3–4 times per week   **TOTAL WORKOUT TIME** > 20 minutes

Level II Exercise Explanations

The exercises in Level II build on the strength you established in Level I, or on the strength you already had before reading this book. Be sure to check out the Placement Test on page 86 to see if you're ready for Level II. In this level, we continue to work on building strength in the posterior (back) muscles of the body, but now we also start to incorporate a few balance and stabilization exercises as well as exercises that work the entire core musculature.

Level II also introduces a few exercises that fall into the category of "open chain," which means that both feet and/or both hands are not on the ground at all times. By performing open-chain exercises, your body will be forced to stabilize itself so that you don't fall over—just like when you are riding out of the saddle and the left side of your body has to react every time you push your right foot down and vice versa. By teaching the body to efficiently and quickly stabilize itself when one foot or hand is lifted off the ground, you are essentially decreasing your chance of injury, not to mention increasing your confidence and sense of safety on the bike. Have you ever crashed or run into the rider beside you while reaching for your water bottle? That happened because your stabilization wasn't quite up to snuff. Don't worry, Exercise 11 will fix that embarrassing faux pas in no time!

LEVEL II EXERCISES

EXERCISE NUMBER		EXERCISE NAME	MUSCLES TARGETED
1		Opposite Arm/Leg Reach from Plank Position	Low back, glute major
2		Supermans with Heel Touches	Low back, glute major, hamstrings
3		Prone Snow Angels with Shoulder Press	Low back, mid back, upper back, shoulders, lateral hip muscles
4		Walking Hip Bridge	Low back, glutes, hamstrings
5		Shoulder Blade Squeeze from Push-up Position	Mid back
6		Tim-berrr!	Transversus abdominis (TVA)
7		Reverse Crunch	Transversus abdominis (TVA)
8		Seated Boat Row	Obliques

Continued on next page »

LEVEL II EXERCISES (Continued)

EXERCISE NUMBER		EXERCISE NAME	MUSCLES TARGETED
9		Side Plank	Obliques
10		Crossover Squats	Glutes, hamstrings, quads, lateral hip muscles
11		Grab the Water Bottle	Transversus abdominis (TVA), shoulder complex, spinal stabilizers
12		The Wall	Transversus abdominis (TVA), shoulder complex, spinal stabilizers
13		TT Position Acceleration	Entire core musculature
14		Overhead Squats	Entire core musculature
15		TT Final Sprint	Entire core musculature

1 ▸ OPPOSITE ARM/LEG REACH FROM PLANK POSITION

GOAL > Improve intramuscular coordination between the core and the extremities; teach the core to use the glute major for hip extension; challenge balance.

Start in a basic TT Hold position by coming onto your forearms and toes, making sure that your elbows are directly below your shoulders and your feet are approximately 10 to 12 inches apart Ⓐ.

Keep your hips and shoulders parallel to the ground and lift your left foot and right hand at the same time Ⓑ. Extend the fingertips forward and toes backward as far as possible. Squeeze your left glute.

Hold this extension for 5 seconds, then bring your hand and foot down to the ground at the same time.

Repeat on the other side Ⓒ and continue alternating until you have completed the designated number of repetitions.

MUSCLES TARGETED

Low back, glute major

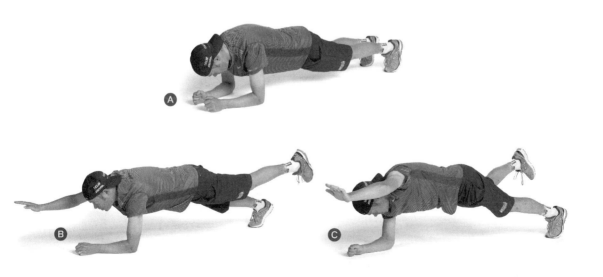

2 | SUPERMANS WITH HEEL TOUCHES

GOAL > Increase strength and range of motion in the low back; teach glutes and hamstrings to fire during hip extension.

Start facedown on the ground with arms extended above your head. Put space between your ears and your shoulders by dropping your shoulder blades down your back.

Gently squeeze your glutes and slowly begin to raise your feet and hands off the ground. Do not lift more than 6 inches. Think about pulling the top of your head and your tailbone in opposite directions.

From this raised position, bend your left leg to a 90-degree angle and reach back with your left hand to touch your left heel Ⓐ.

Return to the superman position (do not relax back down to the ground), and perform the heel touch on the right side Ⓑ. Keep alternating sides until you have completed the designated number of repetitions.

MUSCLES TARGETED

Low back, glute major, hamstrings

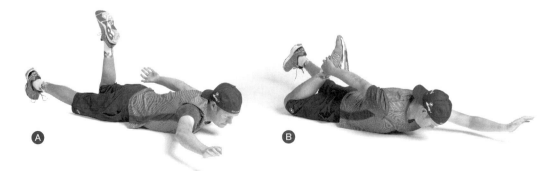

Ⓐ   Ⓑ

3 ❯ PRONE SNOW ANGELS WITH SHOULDER PRESS

GOAL ❯ Increase strength and range of motion in the muscles of the back; teach stabilization in the thoracic and cervical spine when the arms are moving.

Start on the ground in a prone (facedown) position. Start with your arms extended along your sides (palms down), back of the neck long, and shoulder blades dropped down A.

Gently squeeze your glutes and slowly begin to raise your feet, chest, and hands off the ground. Do not lift more than 6 inches.

Create a "snow angel" by sweeping your arms overhead and separating your feet B. Without bending your arms, try to bring your thumbs to touch above your head.

With your hands and feet still lifted, drop your shoulder blades down your back and pull your elbows down to your sides, so that your thumbs eventually touch the tops of your shoulders C.

Push your arms back out straight overhead D and sweep them back down to your sides. Return to starting position by allowing your feet, chest, and hands to relax down to the ground. Continue until you have completed the designated number of repetitions.

If your shoulders and chest muscles are tight, you will not be able to touch your thumbs together above your head. It's better to keep your arms straight and have your hands slightly separated above your head than to bend your arms and touch your thumbs.

MUSCLES TARGETED

Low back, mid back, upper back

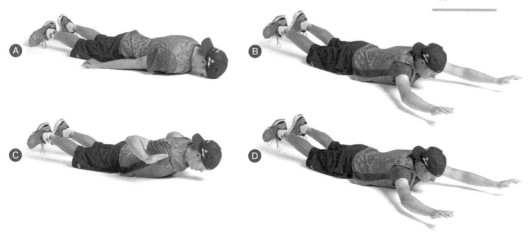

4 | WALKING HIP BRIDGE

GOAL > Release chronic tightness on the front side of the body; teach the glutes and hamstrings to fire during hip extension; increase stabilization in the hips.

Begin by lying on your back with your knees bent and feet on the ground approximately 6 to 8 inches from your glutes A. Squeeze your glutes, tuck your tailbone, and lift your hips off the ground B.

Keeping your hips high and your knees 6 to 8 inches apart, gently lift one knee toward the ceiling and then the other in a "marching"

fashion C D. Although you are marching, try to set each foot down on the ground gently instead of letting the feet stomp.

Throughout the exercise, try to avoid letting the hip rock or sway side to side. Alternate back and forth between your feet until you have completed the designated number of repetitions.

MUSCLES TARGETED

Low back, glutes, hamstring

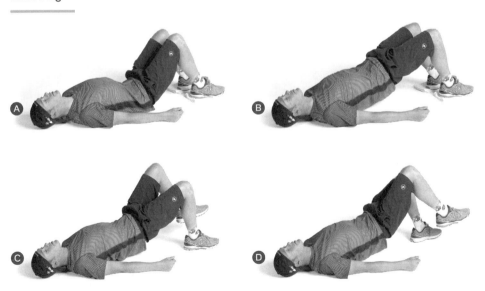

5 ▸ SHOULDER BLADE SQUEEZE FROM PUSH-UP POSITION

GOAL > Combat the cycling slouch; open up the chest cavity to facilitate better breathing; improve shoulder stabilization.

This exercise begins in a push-up position. Place your hands directly below your shoulders and your feet 10 to 12 inches apart Ⓐ.

Keeping your arms straight, drop your shoulder blades down toward your back, then squeeze them together Ⓑ. Don't let your low back sway or your chin push forward.

Hold the shoulder blade squeeze for the designated amount of time and release.

MUSCLES TARGETED

Mid back

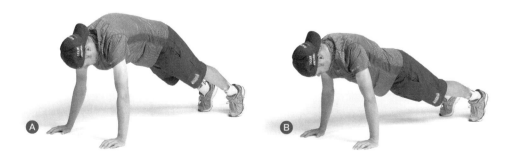

6 TIM-BERRR!

GOAL > Improve activation of the transversus abdominis muscles (TVA); decrease chronic pain in the low back.

We jokingly named this exercise Tim-berrr!, because the way the legs are lowered toward the ground reminds us of a tree falling. The goal is to keep the legs totally straight while they are "falling," mimicking a tree.

Start on your back and extend both legs straight up to the ceiling A. Gently pull your toes toward your face so that the bottoms of your feet are perfectly flat. If your hamstrings are tight, you might need to bend your knees slightly.

Keep your left leg straight while you lower your right leg B until the right heel taps the floor C. Try not to bend your right leg while you are lowering it.

Using your lower abdominals, pull your right leg back up to the starting position, being careful to keep your upper body, neck, and head relaxed the entire time.

Repeat this movement with left leg, and continue to alternate until you have completed the designated number of repetitions.

MUSCLES TARGETED

Transversus
abdominis

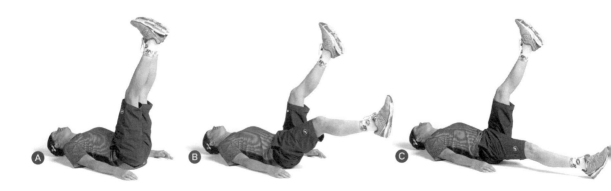

7 REVERSE CRUNCH

GOAL > Improve activation of the transversus abdominis muscles (TVA); teach controlled deceleration in all the abdominal muscles.

Start in a regular crunch position on the ground: Lie on your back with your knees bent, feet planted on the ground, hip distance apart and approximately 6 to 8 inches away from your glutes .

Keeping your upper body completely relaxed, engage the TVA and lift your knees in toward your chest **B**. Think of rolling one vertebra at a time off the ground and then return to the starting position by placing one vertebra down on the ground at a time. Continue until you have completed the designated number of repetitions.

MUSCLES TARGETED

Transversus abdominis

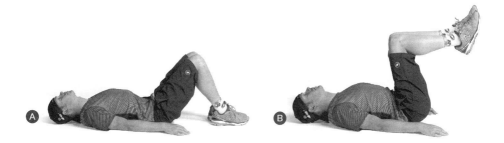

8 | SEATED BOAT ROW

GOAL > Improve rotational strength and stabilization in the obliques; teach chest not to collapse during torso rotation.

Start in a seated position on a mat or carpet with your knees bent and heels lightly touching the ground. Lift your chest, pull your shoulder blades down and together, and keep your neck neutral.

Hold an imaginary oar in front of you with both hands and slowly begin to lean backward until you feel your abdominal muscles start to shake A. Keep your chest lifted and don't round your shoulders. From your shaking position, begin to paddle on either side of your body B C with your imaginary oar until you have completed the designated number of repetitions.

MUSCLES TARGETED

Obliques

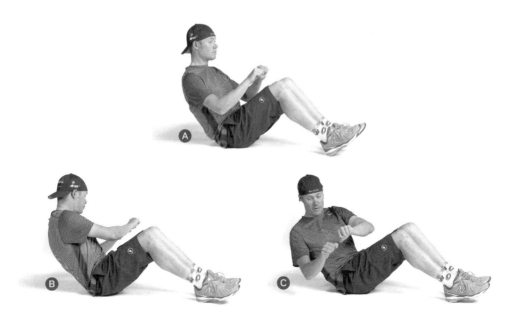

9 ▷ SIDE PLANK

GOAL > Improve muscular strength and activation of the internal obliques.

Remember those irksome side planks from Level I? Now your training wheels get taken away, and you have to complete the exercise without your bottom knee on the ground.

Begin by lying on your right side with your right forearm on the ground, keeping your right elbow directly below your right shoulder Ⓐ. Keep your legs straight, stack your feet, and create a straight line from your left shoulder all the way down to your left ankle. Check to make sure your hips are pushed forward, tailbone is tucked, and your ears are directly above your shoulders.

Place your left hand on your hip, or if you need some extra stability, you can place it on the floor in front of your chest. Push down through the right forearm and lift your hips off the ground Ⓑ. The goal is to get the left side of the hip as far off the ground as possible.

Switch sides and repeat until you have completed the designated number of repetitions.

MUSCLES TARGETED

Obliques

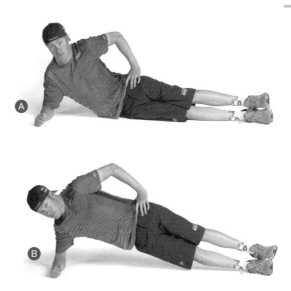

10 CROSSOVER SQUATS

GOAL > Teach the glute medius and lateral hip musculature to stabilize the pelvis in the sagittal plane (side to side).

Start in a standing position with feet hip-distance apart and hands on hips, using good posture in the upper body A. Without bending forward at the waist, step the right foot behind the left at a 45-degree angle off the left heel.

Work to bend both knees as much as possible, but do not go lower than a 90-degree angle at the knee joint B.

Return to standing position C, and repeat the designated number of repetitions on this side before switching to the other foot D.

MUSCLES TARGETED

Glutes, hamstrings, quads, lateral hip muscles

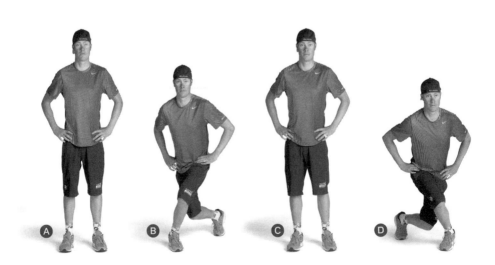

A   B   C   D

11 ▷ GRAB THE WATER BOTTLE

GOAL > Increase dynamic balance and stabilization in the core while the upper body is moving.

We've all done it: a nice, easy descent on a 5 percent grade. That's a great time to grab a quick drink before you start climbing again. You take your right hand off the handlebars and reach down to grab your bottle but can't seem to connect with it on the first try. You take your eyes off the road for less than a second to look down and locate the bottle, and when you look back up you have veered 10 feet to the left and are about to run into oncoming traffic. Time to work on balance and stabilization!

Start in a push-up position with your hands directly below your shoulders, feet 8 to 10 inches apart, and tailbone slightly tucked A.

Slowly and with control, lift your right hand off the ground and begin to reach under your body toward your left foot, as if you were going to grab a water bottle B.

Return your right hand to the ground C, and switch to the left hand D. Keep alternating until you have completed the designated number of repetitions.

The goal is to avoid any rocking in the hips and shoulders while you are moving your arm. Try the first half of the set without moving your head and neck then do the second half with your eyes following your hand while it reaches down.

MUSCLES TARGETED

Transversus abdominis, shoulder complex, spinal stabilizers

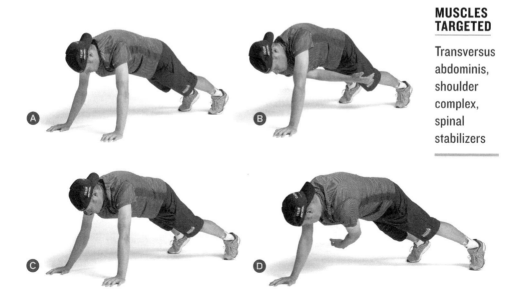

12 > THE WALL

GOAL > Increase dynamic balance and stabilization in the core while the lower body is moving.

Cyclists frequently call a long, steep climb "the Wall" because it challenges the muscles, the endurance, and the brain. The same goes for this exercise, but when you're done you will also have that same exhilarating feeling of accomplishment.

Start in a push-up position with your hands directly below your shoulders, feet 8 to 10 inches apart, and tailbone slightly tucked A.

Slowly and with control, lift your left foot off the ground and bend your left knee in toward your left elbow B. Keep your shoulders and hips quiet and parallel with the ground.

Return your left foot to the starting position and switch legs C. Continue switching legs until you have completed the designated number of repetitions.

This exercise can also be performed from a plank position (forearms on the ground) if you need more stabilization.

MUSCLES TARGETED

Transversus abdominis, shoulder complex, spinal stabilizers

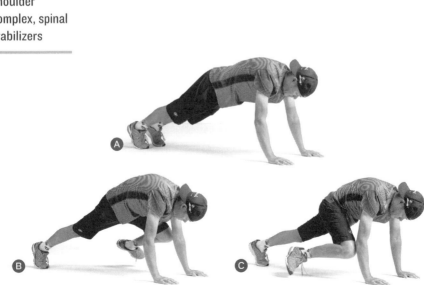

13 ▸ TT (TIME TRIAL) POSITION ACCELERATION

GOAL > Engage all the muscles of the core equally; improve intramuscular coordination among the upper back, lower back, and lower abs.

You mastered the TT Position Hold in Level I, and now it's time to start "pedaling" toward the finish line.

Start with the basic TT Position Hold on your forearms and toes Ⓐ. Elbows should be directly beneath your shoulders, and your feet should be 8 to 10 inches apart.

Keep the back of your neck long and do not look up or down. Work to bring your shoulder blades onto your back by squeezing them together slightly; your upper back should not be rounded. Your lower back should not be

excessively rounded either, nor should you adopt a swayback position.

Keeping your shoulders and hips quiet and parallel to the ground, slowly drop your right knee to the ground without allowing your hips to move or sway Ⓑ. Bring your right knee back to the starting position and drop your left knee Ⓒ.

Continue alternating knees until you have completed the designated number of repetitions.

MUSCLES TARGETED

Entire core musculature

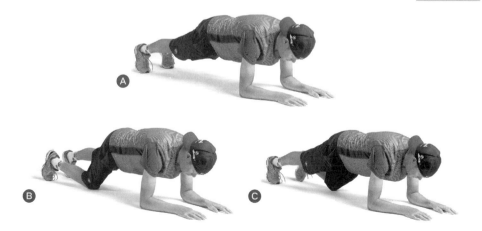

14 ▸ OVERHEAD SQUATS

GOAL > Improve the ability of the core to support the entire spinal column during movement; teach the glutes and hamstrings to fire so the quads aren't overworked.

The overhead squat is used by exercise scientists everywhere as a way to diagnose postural distortions and faulty movement patterns in the body. The overhead squat requires the major muscle groups of the lower body, core, and upper body to work simultaneously. If there is a faulty muscle-firing pattern in one part of the body, it will be revealed at the point of origin and also at various points up and down the kinetic chain.

Start in a standing position with your feet hip-distance apart Ⓐ. Reach both arms up to the ceiling and do not bend at the elbows Ⓑ. Engage the TVA muscle by dropping your tailbone and pulling the lower abdominals toward your spine.

Keeping your core engaged, slowly come into a squat position by pushing your buttocks back first, then lowering them toward the ground Ⓒ. Keep the majority of your body weight in your heels and do not let your knees push forward beyond your toes. Return to the starting position and repeat until you have completed the designated number of repetitions.

If you find yourself shifting weight into your toes and letting your arms fall forward, try performing this exercise with a chair behind you.

MUSCLES TARGETED

Entire core musculature

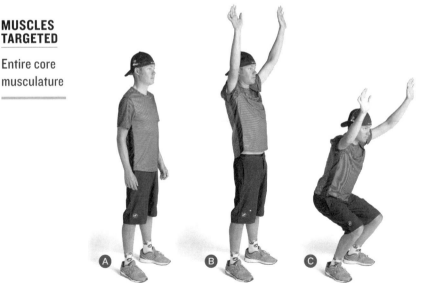

15 ‣ TT (TIME TRIAL) FINAL SPRINT

GOAL > Engage the entire core musculature in a position similar to being on a bike.

It's the final kilometer of a time trial (or maybe the Saturday group ride with your buddies), and you dig deep to finish out the ride strongly. Every muscle in your core is contracted and holding on for dear life, while your arms start to push the handlebars forward. This exercise will help you extract every ounce of strength and stamina by teaching your core to hold still while your arms are sliding back and forth.

Grab two small hand towels for this exercise. Begin in the basic TT Hold position with one towel under each elbow .

Without moving your lower body or rocking your hips, slowly slide your right forearm forward 3 inches while pulling your left forearm back 3 inches (B).

Continue to slide your forearms back and forth, being sure to keep the rest of the body as still as possible (C).

MUSCLES TARGETED

Entire core musculature

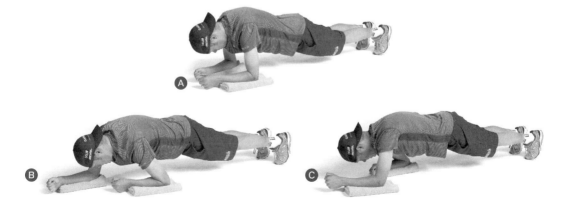

CHAPTER 8

Level III Workouts and Exercises

If you are ready for Level III, you have either successfully made it through at least four weeks each of the Level I and Level II core strength routines in this book, or you already have killer core strength. In the latter case, be sure to check the Placement Test on page 86 to make sure you are ready for these; they are more challenging than they may at first appear.

Level III offers five routines that require a high level of neuromuscular control, endurance, and power. The dynamic warm-up exercises at this level are the same as in the earlier levels, but the exercises in the workout portion are much more challenging, the total volume of sets and reps is higher, the tempo is a bit quicker, and the rest time is shorter. In other words, it's time to play.

It might seem unusual to still include a Workout 1: Injury Prevention/Rehab workout at this level, but many accomplished cyclists need to have this type of routine to fall back on if they have an injury in the middle of the season. This is the only workout in Level III where the tempo is slower and the rest period longer, both of which allow you to concentrate on supporting your joints and allowing the correct muscles to fire.

Workout 2: Posture Correction is a type of routine that Level III cyclists tend to loathe, yet it is very necessary. After all, some of the best cyclists in the world are walking around with horrible posture. The harsh reality is that the sport of cycling requires the body to maintain poor posture for hours on end, and if you are committed to becoming a better cyclist, you are essentially committed to a lifetime of combating poor posture. When Tommy returns from a summer of racing in Europe, he always starts his off-season training with Workout 2.

The routine for Workout 3: Stability and Bike Handling is extremely challenging. It is meant to mimic treacherous riding and racing conditions that require quick reaction times and the ability to maintain control of the bike regardless of external forces. In this routine you will see three exercises for balance and stabilization and three for the entire core.

Workout 4: Endurance is the longest routine in all of the levels. You will be asked to complete 3 sets of each exercise with very little rest between sets. As an additional challenge, the number of repetitions has been increased to 20 on a few of the exercises. Although increasing your time to fatigue is the ultimate goal here, don't sacrifice form in order to complete the workout. It is always better to complete 12 reps with great form than 20 reps with poor form.

Workout 5 in Level III is the ultimate performance-enhancing core strength routine. If you can make it through this workout with good form, you have truly achieved optimum core strength. Now take that fitness and go kick some butt on your rides!

TOMMY'S TAKE

One of my strengths is climbing out of the saddle. When I noticed some areas in my technique that could use some improvement, I took these concerns to Allison and asked her to customize an exercise that would help me accelerate better out of the saddle. She came up with the exercise we named "Musette" that you see here in Level III, which helps to improve strength in the internal obliques while the body is in a balancing position—exactly what I need when I'm out of the saddle. After only a few weeks with this new exercise, I could see a direct improvement in my climbing technique!

LEVEL III, WORKOUT 1	INJURY-PREVENTION/REHAB WORKOUT

GOAL > To decrease pain, increase neuromuscular efficiency, and address long-standing muscular imbalances that cause injury.

TYPE	EXERCISE	MUSCLES TARGETED	SETS	REPS	TEMPO	REST
DYNAMIC WARM-UP	Low-Back Stretch in Doorway (p. 80)	Low back, obliques	I	3 up and down each side	3/3	None
	Rainbow Stretch in Doorway (p. 82)	Obliques, lats, shoulders, lateral hip muscles	I	10 each side	3/3	None
	Supine Figure 4 (p. 83)	Low back, glutes, lateral hip muscles	I	10 each leg	2/2	None
WORKOUT	Opposite Arm/ Leg Reach from Push-up Position (p. 157)	Low back, mid back, upper back, glute major	3	10 each side	I/I	30 seconds
	Back Extension with Hands Under Chin (p. 158)	Low back, mid back, upper back	3	15	2/2	30 seconds
	Inchworms (p. 161)	Transversus abdominis (TVA)	3	15	2/2	30 seconds
	Tick-Tocks (p. 165)	Abdominal muscles, lateral hip muscles	3	10 each leg	I/I	30 seconds

FREQUENCY > 3–5 times per week   **TOTAL WORKOUT TIME** > 18 minutes

LEVEL III, WORKOUT 2 > POSTURE-CORRECTION WORKOUT

GOAL > To correct muscular tightness and weakness, improve joint mobility, and establish optimum positioning of the spinal column.

TYPE	EXERCISE	MUSCLES TARGETED	SETS	REPS	TEMPO	REST
DYNAMIC WARM-UP	Kneeling Quad to Hamstring Stretch (p. 79)	Quads, hamstrings, glutes, calves	1	10 each leg	3/3	None
	Chest Stretch Against Wall (p. 81)	Shoulders, chest	1	10 each arm	3/3	None
	Rainbow Stretch in Doorway (p. 82)	Obliques, lats, shoulders, lateral hip muscles	1	10 each side	3/3	None
WORKOUT	Opposite Arm/ Leg Reach from Push-up Position (p. 157)	Low back, mid back, upper back, glute major	3	10 each side	1/1	30 seconds
	Windshield Wipers (p. 159)	Low back, mid back, glutes, obliques	3	15	2/2	30 seconds
	Jackknives (p. 160)	Transversus abdominis (TVA)	3	15	2/2	30 seconds
	Musette (p. 164)	Obliques	3	10 each side	1/1	30 seconds
	Toss the Water Bottle (p. 171)	Entire core musculature	3	10 each side	1/1	30 seconds

FREQUENCY > 3–5 times per week   **TOTAL WORKOUT TIME** > 22 minutes

LEVEL III, WORKOUT 3	STABILITY AND BIKE-HANDLING WORKOUT

GOAL > To improve static and dynamic stabilization of the entire core musculature, increase muscle-firing efficiency, and improve intramuscular coordination.

TYPE	EXERCISE	MUSCLES TARGETED	SETS	REPS	TEMPO	REST
DYNAMIC WARM-UP	Low-Back Stretch in Doorway (p. 80)	Low back, obliques	1	10 each side	3/3	None
	Chest Stretch Against Wall (p. 81)	Shoulders, chest	1	10 each arm	3/3	None
	Rainbow Stretch in Doorway (p. 82)	Obliques, lats, shoulders, lateral hip muscles	1	10 each side	3/3	None
WORKOUT	Competition Check (p. 166)	Obliques, low back, transversus abdominis (TVA)	3	10 each side	1/1	30 seconds
	Single-Leg Dead Lifts (p. 167)	Glute complex, hamstrings, low back	3	10 each side	2/2	30 seconds
	Single-Leg Squats (p. 168)	Glute complex, hamstrings, quads	3	10 each leg	2/2	30 seconds
	Oblique Crossovers (p. 169)	Entire core musculature	3	10 each side	1/1	30 seconds
	Jumping Jacks on the Floor (p. 170)	Entire core musculature	3	15	As fast as possible	30 seconds

FREQUENCY > 2–3 times per week　　　　**TOTAL WORKOUT TIME** > 22 minutes

LEVEL III, WORKOUT 4 > ENDURANCE WORKOUT

GOAL > To improve muscular endurance and efficiency of the core, and increase time to exhaustion.

TYPE	EXERCISE	MUSCLES TARGETED	SETS	REPS	TEMPO	REST
DYNAMIC WARM-UP	Kneeling Quad to Hamstring Stretch (p. 79)	Quads, hamstrings, glutes, calves	1	10 each leg	3/3	None
	Chest Stretch Against Wall (p. 81)	Shoulders, chest	1	10 each arm	3/3	None
	Rainbow Stretch in Doorway (p. 82)	Obliques, lats, shoulders, lateral hip muscles	1	10 each side	3/3	None
WORKOUT	Back Extension with Hands Under Chin (p. 158)	Low back, mid back, upper back	3	15	1/1	15 seconds
	Inchworms (p. 161)	Transversus abdominis (TVA)	3	15	2/2	15 seconds
	Side Plank with Hip Drops (p. 163)	Obliques, lateral hip muscles	3	15 each side	1/1	15 seconds
	Musette (p. 164)	Obliques	3	15 each side	1/1	15 seconds
	Single-Leg Dead Lifts (p. 167)	Glute complex, hamstrings, low back	3	15 each leg	2/2	15 seconds
	Oblique Crossovers (p. 169)	Entire core musculature	3	15 each leg	1/1	15 seconds

FREQUENCY > 2–3 times per week   **TOTAL WORKOUT TIME** > 27 minutes

LEVEL III, WORKOUT 5 ⟩ TOMMY D'S OPTIMUM PERFORMANCE WORKOUT

GOAL > To develop optimum core strength, increase power production, improve muscular endurance, and be able to keep up with Tom while he climbs Alpe d'Huez.

TYPE	EXERCISE	MUSCLES TARGETED	SETS	REPS	TEMPO	REST
DYNAMIC WARM-UP	Low-Back Stretch in Doorway (p. 80)	Low back, obliques	I	3 each side	3/3	None
	Rainbow Stretch in Doorway (p. 82)	Obliques, lats, shoulders, lateral hip muscles	I	10 each side	3/3	None
	Supine Figure 4 (p. 83)	Low back, glutes, lateral hip muscles	I	10 each leg	3/3	None
WORKOUT	Jackknives (p. 160)	Transversus abdominis (TVA)	3	10	2/2	30 seconds
	Bicycle Crunch (p. 162)	Obliques, rectus abdominis, transversus abdominis	3	10 each side	I/I	30 seconds
	Competition Check (p. 166)	Obliques, low back, transversus abdominis (TVA)	3	10 each side	I/I	30 seconds
	Single-Leg Squats (p. 168)	Glute complex, hamstrings, quads	3	10 each leg	2/2	30 seconds
	Jumping Jacks on the Floor (p. 170)	Entire core musculature	3	30	As fast as possible	30 seconds

FREQUENCY > 3–4 times per week   **TOTAL WORKOUT TIME** > 23 minutes

Level III Exercise Explanations

If you've made it to Level III, you've been working hard on building a strong, powerful core, and you're ready to take that strength to the next level of efficiency and performance. You can still work on addressing postural issues and nagging injuries in Level III, but you will do so with exercises that require more neuromuscular competence than was required in Levels I and II. The obliques are also worked a bit more in Level III, which is a reflection of the fact that your spine is ready to handle more twisting and to move through a greater range of motion.

In general, the goal of Level III is to work your core in a manner that mimics movements performed on the bike. At this point you already know how to activate your TVA and stabilize your entire body with only one hand or foot on the ground; because of this, the exercises in this level will force you to engage multiple muscles and joints throughout different planes of motion. Being a successful cyclist requires you to react quickly and to recruit the correct muscles to perform movements without thinking. The exercises in Level III will help you establish this type of split-second performance with the muscles of the core, which will help make you a better cyclist, decrease your chances of injury, and increase your overall butt-kicking ability.

LEVEL III EXERCISES

EXERCISE NUMBER		EXERCISE NAME	MUSCLES TARGETED
1		Opposite Arm/Leg Reach from Push-up Position	Low back, mid back, upper back, glute major
2		Back Extension with Hands Under Chin	Low back, mid back, upper back
3		Windshield Wipers	Low back, glutes, obliques
4		Jackknives	Transversus abdominis (TVA)
5		Inchworms	Transversus abdominis (TVA)
6		Bicycle Crunch	Obliques, rectus abdominis, transversus abdominis
7		Side Plank with Hip Drops	Obliques, lateral hip muscles
8		Musette	Obliques

Continued on next page »

LEVEL III EXERCISES (Continued)

EXERCISE NUMBER		EXERCISE NAME	MUSCLES TARGETED
9		Tick-Tocks	Abdominal muscles, lateral hip muscles
10		Competition Check	Obliques, low back, transversus abdominis (TVA)
11		Single-Leg Dead Lifts	Glute complex, hamstrings, low back
12		Single-Leg Squats	Glute complex, hamstrings, quads
13		Oblique Crossovers	Entire core musculature
14		Jumping Jacks on the Floor	Entire core musculature
15		Toss the Water Bottle	Entire core musculature

1 ❭ OPPOSITE ARM/LEG REACH FROM PUSH-UP POSITION

GOAL > Improve intramuscular coordination between the core and the extremities; teach the core to use the glute major for hip extension; create dynamic stabilization throughout the entire spinal column.

Start in a push-up position with your hands directly below your shoulders, feet 8 to 10 inches apart, and tailbone slightly tucked Ⓐ. Keep your hips and shoulders parallel to the ground and lift your right foot and left hand at the same time Ⓑ.

Extend your left fingertips forward and right toes backward as far as possible. Squeeze your right glute. Bring your hand and foot down to the ground at the same time.

Repeat on the other side Ⓒ, and continue alternating until you have completed the designated number of repetitions.

MUSCLES TARGETED

Low back, mid back, upper back, glute major

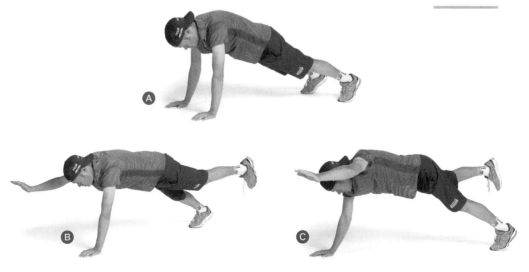

2 BACK EXTENSION WITH HANDS UNDER CHIN

GOAL > Increase strength and range of motion along the entire spinal column.

The back extension is very similar to the Supermans you saw in Levels I and II, but this version calls for your hands to be under your chin.

Lie facedown on the ground and bring both hands under your chin, with your elbows out wide like chicken wings Ⓐ. Put space between your ears and your shoulders by dropping your shoulder blades down toward your waist.

Gently squeeze your glutes and slowly begin to raise your feet and upper body off the ground Ⓑ.

Keep your hands connected to your chin the entire time, but do not crunch the back of your neck upward. Think about pulling the top of your head and your tailbone in opposite directions. As soon as you reach the top of this position (approximately 6 to 8 inches off the ground) slowly lower back down to the ground.

Refresh your starting position each time by dropping your shoulder blades down the back before you lift. Continue until you have completed the designated number of repetitions.

MUSCLES TARGETED

Low back, mid back, upper back

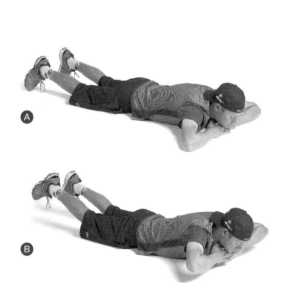

3 WINDSHIELD WIPERS

GOAL > Increase strength and range of motion in the low back; teach obliques and glutes to lift the legs instead of using momentum.

We saw a version of this in Level I, Number II: Supine Knee Drops. In that version, the knees are bent and the emphasis is on the obliques. In this version, the legs are straight, which places greater emphasis on the low back and glutes as well as the obliques.

Begin by lying on your back with your legs straight up in the air, knees and ankles squeezed together. Bring your arms out to a "T" position on the ground with your palms facing down Ⓐ.

Using the pressure of your hands against the ground, slowly begin to drop your legs to the left in a windshield wiper position Ⓑ. Try dropping your legs about I to 2 feet to each side Ⓒ the first time and then slowly begin to work your legs closer to the ground with each repetition Ⓓ.

If your low back begins to act up at all during this exercise, bend your knees in toward your chest.

MUSCLES TARGETED

Low back, glutes, obliques

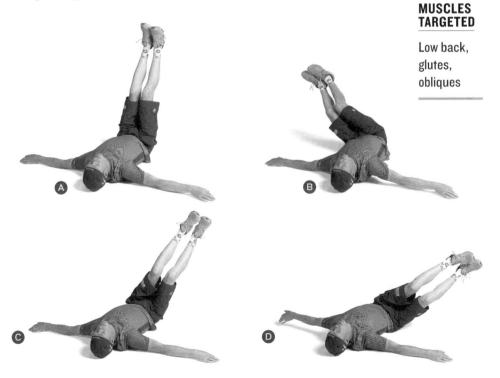

> 4 | JACKKNIVES

GOAL > Increase muscular activation and strength in the TVA; teach the TVA to stabilize the upper body while the legs are moving.

If you've spent much time around springboard divers, you'll recognize this movement. A jackknife is done by touching your toes with your hands, with your hips high up in the air. To facilitate this movement, use two small hand towels, one under each foot.

Start in a push-up position with a small towel under each foot (A). Keep your hands planted, extend your spine long, and slowly begin to slide your feet toward your hands (B). The goal is to keep your legs straight throughout this movement, but if your hamstrings are tight,

you'll need to bend your knees a bit. When you've pulled your feet as close to your hands as possible (C), bend your knees and push your feet back out to the starting position. Continue until you have completed the designated number of repetitions.

A common temptation with this exercise is to "jerk" the feet at the end of the movement to get them closer to the hands. If you are jerking your feet along the ground, you aren't using your core muscles. Keep the movement smooth!

MUSCLES TARGETED

Transversus abdominis

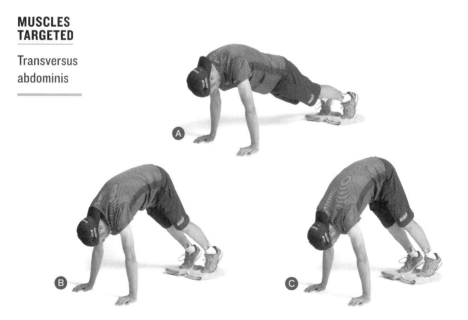

5 INCHWORMS

GOAL > Increase muscular activation and strength in the TVA; teach the TVA to stabilize the lower body while the upper body is moving.

This exercise is similar to the Jackknife, but this time the towels go under the hands instead of the feet.

Start in a push-up position with a small towel under each hand Ⓐ. Keep your hands planted and gently walk your feet as close to your hands as possible Ⓑ, working to keep your legs as straight as your hamstrings will allow Ⓒ.

Using your core, push both hands out at the same time Ⓓ until you reach your starting push-up position Ⓔ. Keep "inchworming" your way along the ground until you have completed the designated number of repetitions.

MUSCLES TARGETED

Transversus abdominis

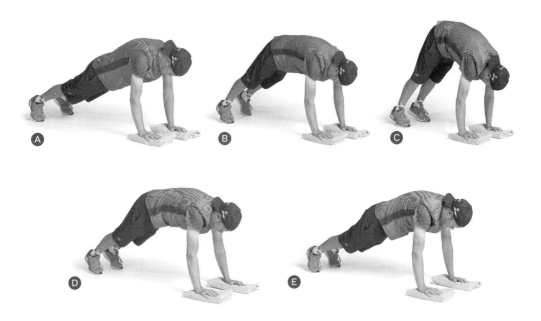

6 BICYCLE CRUNCH

GOAL > Teach the abdominal muscles to work slowly and with control instead of using momentum.

After all that talk in the first part of the book about how you should stop doing crunches, you may be surprised to find a Bicycle Crunch here. If you can complete Level III exercises, you are ready to start learning how to engage your rectus abdominis in a controlled manner. You'll notice that this version of the Bicycle Crunch is performed slowly, which gives the rectus abdominis the opportunity to practice slowing down the extension and rotation of the spine.

Begin by lying on your back with your hands behind your head. Bend your right leg and bring it to a 90-degree angle, with your knee directly above your hip and your right shin parallel to the ground Ⓐ.

Lift your chest toward the ceiling and twist your left elbow toward your right knee, being careful not to bring your right knee closer to your chest; it must remain directly over your right hip Ⓑ.

Keeping your chest lifted, extend your right leg out straight and bring your left leg to a 90-degree angle. Twist your right elbow across toward your left knee Ⓒ.

Continue back and forth, using a very slow, very controlled tempo. Remember, the key is to keep your knees above your hips and bring your elbows toward your knees.

MUSCLES TARGETED

Obliques, rectus abdominis, transversus abdominis

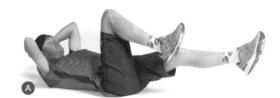

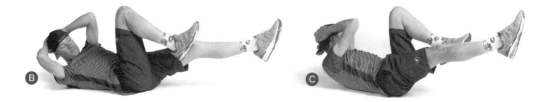

7 | SIDE PLANK WITH HIP DROPS

GOAL > Increase muscular strength and endurance in the obliques and lateral hip muscles.

Start on your right side with your right forearm on the ground, keeping your right elbow directly below your right shoulder. Keep your legs straight, stack your feet, and create a straight line from your left shoulder all the way down to your left ankle. Check to make sure your hips are pushed forward, your tailbone is tucked, and your ears are directly above your shoulders Ⓐ.

Place your left hand on your hip, or if you need some extra stability, you can place it on the floor in front of your chest. Push down through the right forearm and lift your hips off the ground Ⓑ. The goal is to get the left side of the hip as far off the ground as possible.

Lift the hips up and down Ⓒ for the designated number of reps, trying to get the top hip as high as possible with each lift. Finish your set on this side and then switch to the other side.

MUSCLES TARGETED

Obliques, lateral hip muscles

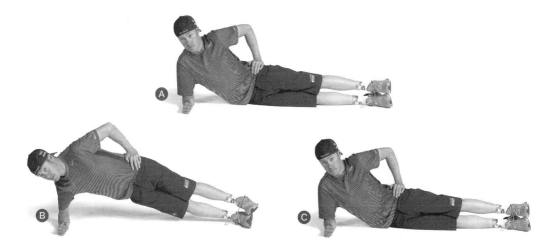

8 ＞ MUSETTE

GOAL > Improve rotational strength and stabilization with an emphasis on the internal obliques; increase strength endurance in the obliques.

This exercise is named after the bags full of food called "musettes" that are given to riders in the feed zone. Riders sling the musettes over one shoulder and then have to sit upright and twist to the side in order to grab the food and fluids inside. Don't go through feed zones very often? This exercise is just as effective for learning how to safely take gels and equipment out of your jersey while riding. Because of the emphasis on the internal obliques, this is also a fabulous exercise for improving rotational stability when riding out of the saddle.

Start in a seated position, your knees bent and heels lightly touching the ground Ⓐ (for a super-advanced option, lift your heels 6 inches off the ground). Lift your chest, pull your

shoulder blades down and together, and keep your neck neutral.

Make a fist with your left hand and push it into your right palm, keeping both hands in the center of your chest and 6 inches away from your body. With your legs held steady, twist your upper body (still pushing that left fist into the right palm) as far to the right as possible Ⓑ.

When you reach your twisting limit, push your left fist into your right hand with as much force as possible for 15 seconds.

Come to center and switch sides, this time, making a fist with your right hand and pushing it into your left palm Ⓒ.

MUSCLES TARGETED

Obliques

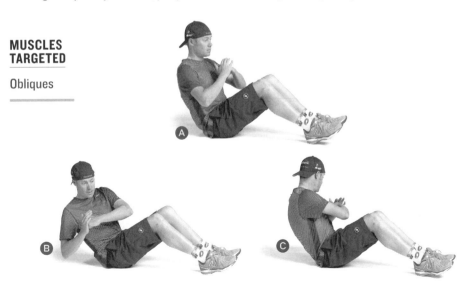

9 TICK-TOCKS

GOAL > Increase muscle activation in the glute medius; teach the core muscles to stabilize the shoulders and hips while the legs are in motion.

Start in a push-up position with a small towel under each foot **A**. Be sure to keep your shoulders directly over your hands and your tailbone slightly tucked.

Without moving your upper body or rocking your hips, slide your left foot 2 to 3 feet out to the left **B**. Keep your toes pointing down

and your left heel pointing directly up to the ceiling.

Slide your left foot back to the starting position and alternate to your right foot **C**. Continue alternating until you have completed the designated number of repetitions.

MUSCLES TARGETED

Abdominal muscles, lateral hip muscles

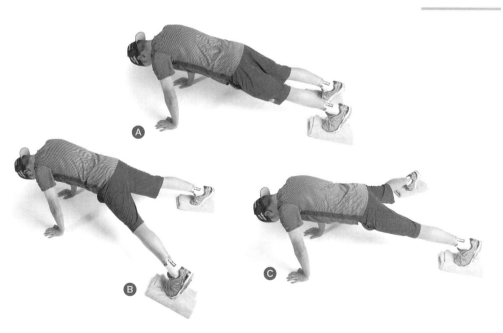

10 > COMPETITION CHECK

GOAL > Improve balance, stabilization, and intramuscular coordination of all the core muscles; decrease risk of crashing when looking over your shoulder.

Have you ever wanted to look behind you on a steep climb to see how much ground you have on your annoying coworker, but you were scared you would lose balance and eat pavement in front of him? This exercise uses almost every muscle of the core, as well as calling upon that large range of motion you've developed from doing dynamic stretches.

Start in a push-up position with your shoulders directly over your hands and your tailbone slightly tucked Ⓐ. Keeping your hips low, pick your right foot up off the ground and start to bring your right knee in toward your right elbow while you simultaneously turn your head to look at your knee Ⓑ Ⓒ. This should create a crunch on the right side of your body.

Return to the starting position and repeat on the right side for the designated number of repetitions, then switch sides.

MUSCLES TARGETED

Obliques, low back, transversus abdominis

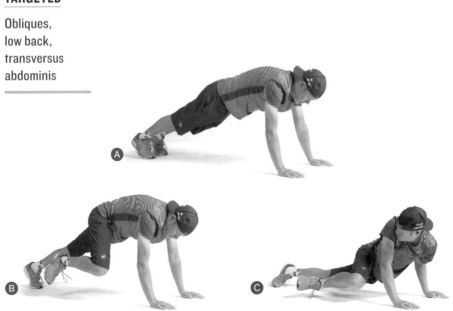

> **11** **SINGLE-LEG DEAD LIFTS**

GOAL > Improve balance and stabilization throughout the entire core musculature; lengthen and strengthen the hamstrings.

Dead Lifts . . . isn't that like an Olympic weight lifting move? Yes, it certainly is, when both legs are on the ground and you're lifting a bar loaded with four times your body weight. However, when dead lifts are performed in a unilateral fashion (one side at a time) with no additional weight, they become an excellent method for working on balance and stability while keeping the core musculature alert and engaged.

Start in a standing position with good posture: tailbone dropped, chest lifted, shoulder blades down and back **A**.

Place your hands on your hips and begin to tilt your upper body forward while lifting your left leg off the ground **B**. The key to a

Single-Leg Dead Lift is to maintain a straight line from the shoulders through the hips and all the way down the leg that is lifted. A common mistake is to bend at the waist, which causes the upper body to drop to the ground, but the leg doesn't lift in back. Think of your torso and your leg as a seesaw; however far down your torso falls, your back leg must lift an equal amount off the ground **C**.

Return to the starting position by simultaneously lifting your chest and lowering your leg, keeping your core engaged the entire time.

Complete the designated number of repetitions on the left; then switch legs and complete the repetitions.

MUSCLES TARGETED

Glute complex, hamstrings, low back

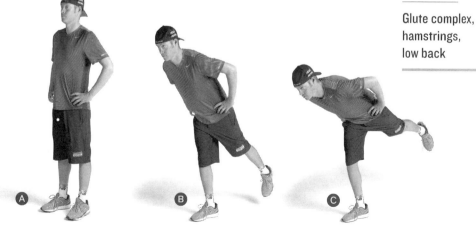

12 > SINGLE-LEG SQUATS

GOAL > Improve the ability of the glute medius to stabilize the femur (thigh bone) in the sagittal plane (side to side); allow the hamstrings to practice deceleration of knee flexion and hip flexion.

Start in a standing position with good posture: tailbone dropped, chest lifted, shoulder blades down and back (A). Place your hands on your hips and lift your right foot 6 to 8 inches off the ground (B).

Shift your weight into the heel of your left foot and begin to push your hips back, then bend your left knee and begin to lower into a squat (C). It is extremely difficult to achieve the same depth with a Single-Leg Squat that you can with a Double-Leg Squat, so be sure to stop as soon as you feel your upper body leaning forward or your knee moving forward over your toes on the supporting leg.

Squeeze the glute on the stabilizing leg as you return to the starting position.

Complete the designated number of repetitions with the right foot lifted, then switch legs and complete the repetitions (D) (E).

MUSCLES TARGETED

Glute complex, hamstrings, quads

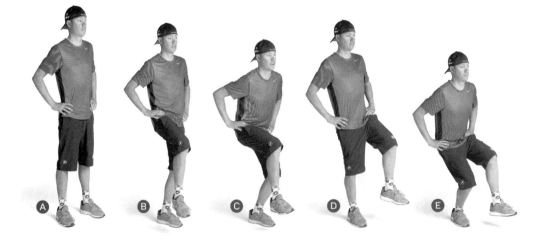

13 ▸ OBLIQUE CROSSOVERS

GOAL > Increase balance and stabilization along the entire spinal column; improve flexibility and range of motion in the lateral hip.

Start in a push-up position with your shoulders directly over your hands and your tailbone slightly tucked Ⓐ.

Keeping your shoulders stable and parallel to the ground, pick up your left leg and begin to pull your left knee under your body toward your right elbow Ⓑ. That's correct; left knee goes to right elbow.

Complete all the repetitions on this side before switching Ⓒ.

For an additional challenge, don't set your foot down on the ground when you extend your leg back out straight. Instead, squeeze the glute and let the foot hover about 6 inches off the ground before pulling the knee back in.

MUSCLES TARGETED

Entire core musculature

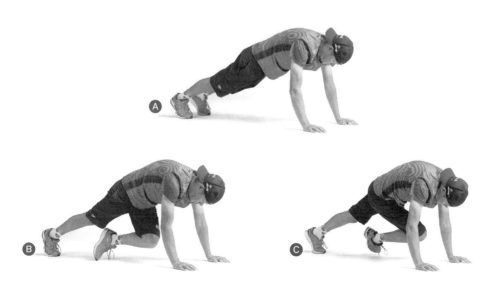

14 JUMPING JACKS ON THE FLOOR

GOAL > Teach the muscles of the core to stabilize the hips and spine during impact.

Start in a TT Hold position with the forearms on the ground Ⓐ. Shoulders should be directly over elbows, neck neutral, tailbone slightly tucked.

Keeping the hips low, jump both feet out at the same time Ⓑ and then both back in Ⓒ, as if

you're doing jumping jacks. The key here is to keep your hips low so your pelvis is supported by the core muscles. Continue until you have completed the designated number of repetitions.

MUSCLES TARGETED

Entire core musculature

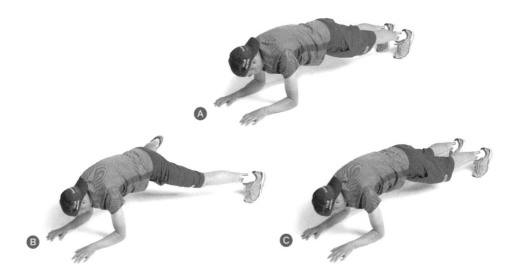

15 ⟩ TOSS THE WATER BOTTLE

GOAL > Challenge the entire core musculature while the upper body, torso, and lower body are all in motion; increase intramuscular coordination throughout the entire body.

Begin by lying on your right side with your right forearm on the ground, keeping your elbow directly below your right shoulder A . Keep your legs straight, stack your feet, and create a straight line from your left shoulder all the way down to your left ankle. Check to make sure your hips are pushed forward, your tailbone is tucked, and your ears are directly above your shoulders.

Lift your hips off the ground, pushing the left as far toward the ceiling as possible B .

Extend your left arm toward the ceiling as well C , and then drop it down under the right side of your body and "thread" it through the space between the ground and the right side of your rib cage D . Then reach your arm back up toward the ceiling C .

Continue this threading motion with your left hand for the designated number of repetitions.

Roll to the other side and repeat.

MUSCLES TARGETED

Entire core musculature

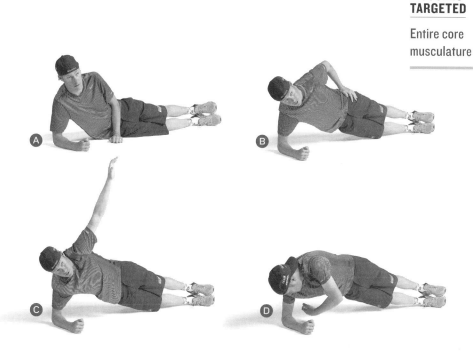

APPENDIX
WORKOUT LOGS

LEVEL I, WORKOUT 1	INJURY PREVENTION/REHAB WORKOUT

GOAL > To decrease pain, increase neuromuscular efficiency, and address long-standing muscular imbalances that cause injury.

TYPE	EXERCISE	SETS	REPS	TEMPO	REST	SETS	REPS	REST
DYNAMIC WARM-UP	Low-Back Stretch in Doorway	I	3 up and down each side	3/3	None			
	Rainbow Stretch in Doorway	I	10 each side	3/3	None			
	Supine Figure 4	I	10 each leg	2/2	None			
WORKOUT	Opposite Arm/Leg Reach	2	10 each side	2/2	30 seconds			
	Hip Bridge with Heel Slides	2	10 each leg	2/2	30 seconds			
	TVA Activation	I	5	Hold 5 seconds	5 seconds between each rep			
	Tailbone Tucks	I	5	Hold 5 seconds	5 seconds between each rep			

FREQUENCY > 3–5 times per week

WEEKS ON PROGRAM > _____   **WORKOUTS COMPLETED THIS WEEK** > _____

NOTES *(how you felt, hardest exercise, noticeable progress, etc.)* > _____

_____

LEVEL I, WORKOUT 2	POSTURE-CORRECTION WORKOUT

GOAL > To correct muscular tightness and weakness, improve joint mobility, and establish optimum positioning of the spinal column.

TYPE	EXERCISE	SETS	REPS	TEMPO	REST	SETS	REPS	REST
DYNAMIC WARM-UP	Kneeling Quad to Hamstring Stretch	1	10 each leg	3/3	None			
	Chest Stretch Against Wall	1	10 each arm	3/3	None			
	Rainbow Stretch in Doorway	1	10 each side	3/3	None			
WORKOUT	Prone Snow Angels	2	15	2/2	30 seconds			
	Shoulder Blade Squeeze	1	10	Hold 5 seconds	5 seconds between each rep			
	TVA Activation	1	10	Hold 5 seconds	5 seconds between each rep			
	Pac-Mans	2	15 each leg	3/3	30 seconds			
	Chair Squats	2	15	2/2	30 seconds			

FREQUENCY > 3–5 times per week

WEEKS ON PROGRAM > _____   **WORKOUTS COMPLETED THIS WEEK >** _____

NOTES *(how you felt, hardest exercise, noticeable progress, etc.)* > _____

LEVEL I, WORKOUT 3 > STABILITY AND BIKE-HANDLING WORKOUT

GOAL > To improve static and dynamic stabilization of the entire core musculature, increase muscle firing efficiency, and improve intramuscular coordination.

TYPE	EXERCISE	SETS	REPS	TEMPO	REST	SETS	REPS	REST
DYNAMIC WARM-UP	Low-Back Stretch in Doorway	1	10 each side	3/3	None			
	Chest Stretch Against Wall	1	10 each arm	3/3	None			
	Rainbow Stretch in Doorway	1	10 each side	3/3	None			
WORKOUT	Supermans	2	12	2/2	30 seconds			
	Mountain Climbers	2	12 each leg	2/2	30 seconds			
	Side Planks	2	12 each side	2/2	30 seconds			
	Audrey Two	2	12 each leg	2/2	30 seconds			
	TT Position Hold	2	1	Hold for 20–30 seconds	30 seconds			

FREQUENCY > 2–3 times per week

WEEKS ON PROGRAM > _____   **WORKOUTS COMPLETED THIS WEEK >** _____

NOTES *(how you felt, hardest exercise, noticeable progress, etc.)* > _____

_____

LEVEL I, WORKOUT 4 — ENDURANCE WORKOUT

GOAL > To improve muscular endurance and efficiency of the core and increase time to exhaustion.

TYPE	EXERCISE	SETS	REPS	TEMPO	REST	SETS	REPS	REST
DYNAMIC WARM-UP	Kneeling Quad to Hamstring Stretch	1	10 each leg	3/3	None			
	Chest Stretch Against Wall	1	10 each arm	3/3	None			
	Rainbow Stretch in Doorway	1	10 each side	3/3	None			
WORKOUT	Hip Bridge with Heel Slides	2	15 each leg	2/2	30 seconds			
	Mountain Climbers	2	15 each leg	2/2	30 seconds			
	Supine Knee Drops	2	15 each side	2/2	30 seconds			
	Pac-Mans	2	15 each leg	2/2	30 seconds			
	TT Position Hold	2	1	Hold 30–40 seconds	30 seconds			

FREQUENCY > 2–3 times per week

WEEKS ON PROGRAM > _____   **WORKOUTS COMPLETED THIS WEEK >** _____

NOTES *(how you felt, hardest exercise, noticeable progress, etc.)* > _____

_____

LEVEL I, WORKOUT 5	TOMMY D'S OPTIMUM PERFORMANCE WORKOUT

GOAL > To develop optimum core strength, increase power production, improve muscular endurance, and be able to keep up with Tom while he climbs Alpe d'Huez.

TYPE	EXERCISE	SETS	REPS	TEMPO	REST	SETS	REPS	REST
DYNAMIC WARM-UP	Low-Back Stretch in Doorway	1	3 each side	3/3	None			
	Rainbow Stretch in Doorway	1	10 each side	3/3	None			
	Supine Figure 4	1	10 each leg	3/3	None			
WORKOUT	Prone Snow Angels	2	12	2/2	30 seconds			
	Hip Bridge with Heel Slides	2	12 each leg	2/2	30 seconds			
	Mountain Climbers	2	12 each leg	2/2	30 seconds			
	Side Planks	2	12 each side	2/2	30 seconds			
	Chair Squats	2	12	2/2	30 seconds			

FREQUENCY > 3–4 times per week

WEEKS ON PROGRAM > _____   **WORKOUTS COMPLETED THIS WEEK** > _____

NOTES (how you felt, hardest exercise, noticeable progress, etc.) > _____

_____

| LEVEL II, WORKOUT 1 | INJURY PREVENTION/REHAB WORKOUT |

GOAL > To decrease pain, increase neuromuscular efficiency, and address long-standing muscular imbalances that cause injury.

TYPE	EXERCISE	SETS	REPS	TEMPO	REST	SETS	REPS	REST
DYNAMIC WARM-UP	Low-Back Stretch in Doorway	1	3 up and down each side	3/3	None			
	Rainbow Stretch in Doorway	1	10 each side	3/3	None			
	Supine Figure 4	1	10 each leg	2/2	None			
WORKOUT	Opposite Arm/Leg Reach from Plank Position	2	10 each side	2/2	30 seconds			
	Walking Hip Bridge	2	10 each leg	2/2	30 seconds			
	Tim-berrr!	2	10 each leg	2/2	30 seconds			
	Reverse Crunch	2	15	2/2	30 seconds			

FREQUENCY > 3–5 times per week

WEEKS ON PROGRAM > _____   **WORKOUTS COMPLETED THIS WEEK > _____**

NOTES (how you felt, hardest exercise, noticeable progress, etc.) > _____

_____

LEVEL II, WORKOUT 2 > POSTURE-CORRECTION WORKOUT

GOAL > To correct muscular tightness and weakness, improve joint mobility, and establish optimum positioning of the spinal column.

TYPE	EXERCISE	SETS	REPS	TEMPO	REST	SETS	REPS	REST
DYNAMIC WARM-UP	Kneeling Quad to Hamstring Stretch	1	10 each leg	3/3	None			
	Chest Stretch Against Wall	1	10 each arm	3/3	None			
	Rainbow Stretch in Doorway	1	10 each side	3/3	None			
WORKOUT	Prone Snow Angels with Shoulder Press	2	10	2/2 for Angel, 1/1 for Press	30 seconds			
	Shoulder Blade Squeeze from Push-up Position	1	15	Hold 5 seconds	5 seconds between each rep			
	Tim-berrr!	2	10 each leg	2/2	30 seconds			
	Crossover Squats	2	10 each leg	1/1	30 seconds			
	TT Position Acceleration	2	10 each leg	1/1	30 seconds			

FREQUENCY > 3–5 times per week

WEEKS ON PROGRAM > _____   **WORKOUTS COMPLETED THIS WEEK** > _____

NOTES (how you felt, hardest exercise, noticeable progress, etc.) > _____

LEVEL II, WORKOUT 3	STABILITY AND BIKE-HANDLING WORKOUT

GOAL > To improve static and dynamic stabilization of the entire core musculature, increase muscle-firing efficiency, and improve intramuscular coordination.

TYPE	EXERCISE	SETS	REPS	TEMPO	REST	SETS	REPS	REST
DYNAMIC WARM-UP	Low-Back Stretch in Doorway	1	10 each side	3/3	None			
	Chest Stretch Against Wall	1	10 each arm	3/3	None			
	Rainbow Stretch in Doorway	1	10 each side	3/3	None			
WORKOUT	Supermans with Heel Touches	2	10 each side	2/2	30 seconds			
	Side Plank	2	10 each side	2/2	30 seconds			
	Crossover Squats	2	10 each leg	1/1	30 seconds			
	Grab the Water Bottle	2	10 each side	2/2	30 seconds			
	The Wall	2	10 each side	2/2	30 seconds			

FREQUENCY > 3–4 times per week

WEEKS ON PROGRAM > _____   **WORKOUTS COMPLETED THIS WEEK > _____**

NOTES *(how you felt, hardest exercise, noticeable progress, etc.)* **> _____**

LEVEL II, WORKOUT 4 > ENDURANCE WORKOUT

GOAL > To improve muscular endurance and efficiency of the core and increase time to exhaustion.

TYPE	EXERCISE	SETS	REPS	TEMPO	REST	SETS	REPS	REST
DYNAMIC WARM-UP	Kneeling Quad to Hamstring Stretch	1	10 each leg	3/3	None			
	Chest Stretch Against Wall	1	10 each arm	3/3	None			
	Rainbow Stretch in Doorway	1	10 each side	3/3	None			
WORKOUT	Walking Hip Bridge	2	15 each leg	2/2	20 seconds			
	Reverse Crunch	2	15	2/2	20 seconds			
	Seated Boat Row	2	1 each side	Hold 15 seconds	20 seconds			
	TT Position Acceleration	2	15 each leg	1/1	20 seconds			
	Overhead Squats	2	15	2/2	20 seconds			

FREQUENCY > 2–3 times per week

WEEKS ON PROGRAM > _____   **WORKOUTS COMPLETED THIS WEEK** > _____

NOTES *(how you felt, hardest exercise, noticeable progress, etc.)* > _____

LEVEL II, WORKOUT 5	TOMMY D'S OPTIMUM PERFORMANCE WORKOUT

GOAL > To develop optimum core strength, increase power production, improve muscular endurance, and be able to keep up with Tom while he climbs Alpe d'Huez.

TYPE	EXERCISE	SETS	REPS	TEMPO	REST	SETS	REPS	REST
DYNAMIC WARM-UP	Low-Back Stretch in Doorway	1	3 each side	3/3	None			
	Rainbow Stretch win Doorway	1	10 each side	3/3	None			
	Supine Figure 4	1	10 each leg	3/3	None			
WORKOUT	Prone Snow Angels with Shoulder Press	2	12	2/2 Angel, 1/1 Press	30 seconds			
	Reverse Crunch	2	12	2/2	30 seconds			
	Seated Boat Row	2	1 each side	Hold 15 seconds each side	30 seconds			
	Crossover Squats	2	12 each side	1/1	30 seconds			
	Grab the Water Bottle	2	12 each side	1/1	30 seconds			
	TT Final Sprint	2	12 each arm	1/1	30 seconds			

FREQUENCY > 3–4 times per week

WEEKS ON PROGRAM > _____   **WORKOUTS COMPLETED THIS WEEK** > _____

NOTES (how you felt, hardest exercise, noticeable progress, etc.) > _____

LEVEL III, WORKOUT 1	INJURY-PREVENTION/REHAB WORKOUT

GOAL > To decrease pain, increase neuromuscular efficiency, and address long-standing muscular imbalances that cause injury.

TYPE	EXERCISE	SETS	REPS	TEMPO	REST	SETS	REPS	REST
DYNAMIC WARM-UP	Low-Back Stretch in Doorway	I	3 up and down each side	3/3	None			
	Rainbow Stretch in Doorway	I	10 each side	3/3	None			
	Supine Figure 4	I	10 each leg	2/2	None			
WORKOUT	Opposite Arm/ Leg Reach from Push-up Position	3	10 each side	I/I	30 seconds			
	Back Extension with Hands Under Chin	3	15	2/2	30 seconds			
	Inchworms	3	15	2/2	30 seconds			
	Tick-Tocks	3	10 each leg	I/I	30 seconds			

FREQUENCY > 3–5 times per week

WEEKS ON PROGRAM > _____   **WORKOUTS COMPLETED THIS WEEK** > _____

NOTES *(how you felt, hardest exercise, noticeable progress, etc.)* > _____

_____

LEVEL III, WORKOUT 2 > POSTURE-CORRECTION WORKOUT

GOAL > To correct muscular tightness and weakness, improve joint mobility, and establish optimum positioning of the spinal column.

TYPE	EXERCISE	SETS	REPS	TEMPO	REST	SETS	REPS	REST
DYNAMIC WARM-UP	Kneeling Quad to Hamstring Stretch	1	10 each leg	3/3	None			
	Chest Stretch Against Wall	1	10 each arm	3/3	None			
	Rainbow Stretch in Doorway	1	10 each side	3/3	None			
WORKOUT	Opposite Arm/ Leg Reach from Push-Up Position	3	10 each side	1/1	30 seconds			
	Windshield Wipers	3	15	2/2	30 seconds			
	Jackknives	3	15	2/2	30 seconds			
	Musette	3	10 each side	1/1	30 seconds			
	Toss the Water Bottle	3	10 each side	1/1	30 seconds			

FREQUENCY > 3–5 times per week

WEEKS ON PROGRAM > _____   **WORKOUTS COMPLETED THIS WEEK >** _____

NOTES *(how you felt, hardest exercise, noticeable progress, etc.)* > _____

LEVEL III, WORKOUT 3	STABILITY AND BIKE-HANDLING WORKOUT

GOAL > To improve static and dynamic stabilization of the entire core musculature, increase muscle-firing efficiency, and improve intramuscular coordination.

TYPE	EXERCISE	SETS	REPS	TEMPO	REST	SETS	REPS	REST
DYNAMIC WARM-UP	Low-Back Stretch in Doorway	1	10 each side	3/3	None			
	Chest Stretch Against Wall	1	10 each arm	3/3	None			
	Rainbow Stretch in Doorway	1	10 each side	3/3	None			
WORKOUT	Competition Check	3	10 each side	1/1	30 seconds			
	Single-Leg Dead Lifts	3	10 each side	2/2	30 seconds			
	Single-Leg Squats	3	10 each leg	2/2	30 seconds			
	Oblique Crossovers	3	10 each side	1/1	30 seconds			
	Jumping Jacks on the Floor	3	15	As fast as possible	30 seconds			

FREQUENCY > 2–3 times per week

WEEKS ON PROGRAM > _____   **WORKOUTS COMPLETED THIS WEEK** > _____

NOTES *(how you felt, hardest exercise, noticeable progress, etc.)* > _____

_____

LEVEL III, WORKOUT 4 〉 ENDURANCE WORKOUT

GOAL > To improve muscular endurance and efficiency of the core, and increase time to exhaustion.

TYPE	EXERCISE	SETS	REPS	TEMPO	REST	SETS	REPS	REST
DYNAMIC WARM-UP	Kneeling Quad to Hamstring Stretch	1	10 each leg	3/3	None			
	Chest Stretch against Wall	1	10 each arm	3/3	None			
	Rainbow Stretch in Doorway	1	10 each side	3/3	None			
WORKOUT	Back Extension with Hands Under Chin	3	15	1/1	15 seconds			
	Inchworms	3	15	2/2	15 seconds			
	Side Plank with Hip Drops	3	15 each side	1/1	15 seconds			
	Musette	3	15 each side	1/1	15 seconds			
	Single-Leg Dead Lifts	3	15 each leg	2/2	15 seconds			
	Oblique Crossovers	3	15 each leg	1/1	15 seconds			

FREQUENCY > 2–3 times per week

WEEKS ON PROGRAM > _____   **WORKOUTS COMPLETED THIS WEEK** > _____

NOTES *(how you felt, hardest exercise, noticeable progress, etc.)* > _____

LEVEL III, WORKOUT 5	TOMMY D'S OPTIMUM PERFORMANCE WORKOUT

GOAL > To develop optimum core strength, increase power production, improve muscular endurance, and be able to keep up with Tom while he climbs Alpe d'Huez.

TYPE	EXERCISE	SETS	REPS	TEMPO	REST	SETS	REPS	REST
DYNAMIC WARM-UP	Low-Back Stretch in Doorway	I	3 each side	3/3	None			
	Rainbow Stretch in Doorway	I	10 each side	3/3	None			
	Supine Figure 4	I	10 each leg	3/3	None			
WORKOUT	Jackknives	3	10	2/2	30 seconds			
	Bicycle Crunch	3	10 each side	1/1	30 seconds			
	Competition Check	3	10 each side	1/1	30 seconds			
	Single-Leg Squats	3	10 each leg	2/2	30 seconds			
	Jumping Jacks on the Floor	3	30	As fast as possible	30 seconds			

FREQUENCY > 3–4 times per week

WEEKS ON PROGRAM > _____   **WORKOUTS COMPLETED THIS WEEK > _____**

NOTES *(how you felt, hardest exercise, noticeable progress, etc.)* **> _____**

_____

SOURCES

Arbitbol, M. M. 1989. "Sacral Curvature and Supine Posture." *American Journal of Physical Anthropology* 80(3): 378–389.

Asplund, C., and P. St. Pierre. 2004. "Knee Pain and Bicycling: Fitting Concepts for Clinicians." *The Physician and Sports Medicine* 32(4): 23–30.

Bandy, W. D., J. M. Irion, and M. Briggler. 1998. "The Effect of Static Stretch and Dynamic Range of Motion Training on the Flexibility of the Hamstring Muscles." *Journal of Orthopaedic and Sports Physical Therapy* 27(4): 295–300.

Barry, P., M. D. Boden, L. Y. Griffin, and W. E. Garret Jr. 2000. "Etiology and Prevention of Noncontact ACL Injury." *The Physician and Sports Medicine* 28(4). Retrieved from http://www.frvbc.com/newsletter/pdf/Etiology%20and%20Prevention%20of%20Noncontact%20ACL%20Injury%20word.pdf

Bergmark, A. 1989. "Stability of the Lumbar Spine: A Study in Mechanical Engineering." *Acta Orthopaedica Scandinavica* 230 (suppl.): 20–24.

Boyle, M. 2004. *Functional Training for Sports: Superior Conditioning for Today's Athlete.* Champaign, IL: Human Kinetics.

———. "Understanding Hip Flexion." July 15, 2006. Retrieved from www.ptonthenet.com.

Church, J. B., M. S. Wiggins, F. M. Moode, and R. Crist. 2001. "Effect of Warm-up and Flexibility Treatments on Vertical Jump Performance." *Journal of Strength and Conditioning Research* 15(3): 332–336.

Clark, M. A. 2000. "An Integrated Approach to Human Movement Science." Thousand Oaks, CA: National Academy of Sports Medicine, 2000.

Clarsen, B., T. Krosshaug, and R. Bahr. 2010. "Overuse Injuries in Professional Road Cyclists." *The American Journal of Sports Medicine* 38: 2494–2501.

Cook, G. 2003. *Athletic Body in Balance: Optimal Movement Skills and Conditioning for Performance.* Champaign, IL: Human Kinetics.

Curry, B. S, D. Chengkalath, G. J. Crouch, M. Romance, and P. J. Manns. 2009. "Acute Effects of Dynamic Stretching, Static Stretching, and Light Aerobic Activity on Muscular Performance in Women." *Journal of Strength and Conditioning Research* 23(6): 1811–1819.

Delavier, F., J-P Clemenceau, and M. Gundill. 2010. *Delavier's Stretching Anatomy.* Champaign, IL: Human Kinetics.

Hodges, P. W., and C. A. Richardson. 1996. "Inefficient Muscular Stabilization of the Lumbar Spine Associated with Low Back Pain: A Motor Control Evaluation of Transversus Abdominis." *Spine* 21(22): 2640–2650.

Huang, L., A. Galinsky, D. H. Gruenfeld, and L. E. Guillory. 2011. "Powerful Postures Versus Powerful Roles: Which Is the Proximate Correlate of Thought and Behavior?" *Psychological Science* 22(1): 95–102.

Kovacs, M. S. 2010. *Dynamic Stretching.* Berkeley, CA: Ulysses Press.

Magnusson, P., and P. Renstrom. 2006. "The European College of Sports Sciences Position Statement: The Role of Stretching Exercises in Sports." *European Journal of Sport Science* 6(2): 87–91.

National Academy of Sports Medicine. "Current Concepts in Flexibility Training." Retrieved from http://www.nasm.org/1/HFPN/Research_Library/CCPs/Current_Concepts_in_Flexibility_Training/

Neumann, D. A. 2002. *Kinesiology of the Musculoskeletal System: Foundations for Physical Rehabilitation.* St. Louis, MO: Mosby.

Powers, C. 2003. "The Influence of Altered Lower Extremity Kinematics on Patella Femoral Joint Dysfunction." *Journal of Orthopaedic and Sports Physical Therapy* 33: 639–646.

Powers, S. K., and E. T. Howley. 2007. *Exercise Physiology: Theory and Application to Fitness and Performance.* 6th ed. New York: McGraw-Hill.

Sahrmann, S. A. 2002. *Diagnosis and Treatment of Movement Impairment Syndromes.* St. Louis, MO: Mosby.

Schulz, S. J., and S. J. Gordon. 2010. "Recreational Cyclists: The Relationship Between Low Back Pain and Training Characteristics." *International Journal of Exercise Science* 3(3): Article 3.

Shrier, I. 2004. "Does Stretching Improve Performance? A Systematic and Critical Review of the Literature." *Clinical Journal of Sport Medicine* 14(5): 267–273.

Shrier, I., and K. Gossal. 2000. "Myths and Truths of Stretching." *The Physician and Sports Medicine* 28: 57–63.

Szadek, K. M., P. van der Wurff, M. W. Zuurmond, and R. S. Perez. 2009. "Diagnostic Validity of Criteria for Sacroiliac Joint Pain: A Systematic Review." *Journal of Pain* 10(4): 354–368.

Verstegen, M., and P. Williams. 2004. *Core Performance: The Revolutionary Workout Program to Transform Your Body and Your Life.* New York: Rodale.

Suggestions for Further Reading

Athletic Body in Balance, Gray Cook

Dynamic Stretching, Mark Kovacs

Get Fast, Selene Yeager

Weight Training for Cyclists: A Total Body Program for Power and Endurance, Ken Doyle and Eric Schmitz

INDEX

ABOUT THE AUTHORS

TOM DANIELSON is one of the world's top professional road cyclists. His career began with Team Mercury in 2002 and continued with Team Saturn, Fassa Bortolo, and Team Discovery. He is currently a member of Garmin-Sharp-Barracuda. Known for his incredible climbing ability and his large lung capacity, "Tommy D" currently holds the record for the fastest ascent of Mt. Washington in New Hampshire and the Mt. Evans Hill Climb in Colorado.

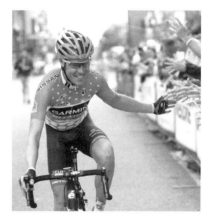

Tom brought home his first major victory, the Dodge Tour de Georgia, in April 2005. The win was sealed on the Brasstown Bald stage, where he left the rest of the peloton gasping and won the stage on the supersteep climb to the finish. Just one year later, while riding for Discovery, Tom won the grueling stage 17 of the Vuelta a España and subsequently supported his team in several victories through 2007. His debut performance in the Tour de France in 2011 resulted in a ninth-place finish, making him the highest-placed American overall. He also led his team to a stage win in the Team Time Trial as well as helping to seal the overall team classification. In 2012, despite having crashed out of the Tour de France just six weeks earlier, Tom once again displayed his fortitude by winning stage 3 of the USA Pro Cycling Challenge, where he was also named Most Aggressive Rider.

In addition to his time in the saddle, Tom is known for his contributions to the sport and his encouragement of young riders. He helped create the Fort Lewis College Cycling Scholarship fund to assist young collegiate cyclists. In November 2006, Tom established the Tom Danielson Junior Race Series and Camps to provide support, encouragement, and skills development to junior racers in a competitive environment.

Tom lives in Boulder with his wife, Stephanie, and their children, Stevie and Stella. He enjoys riding motocross bikes in his spare time.

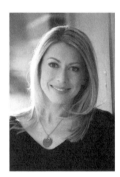

ALLISON WESTFAHL is a nationally renowned exercise physiologist, author, and fitness personality. After graduating magna cum laude from Yale, Allison moved to Colorado to pursue a career in fitness. At the age of 25, she became the youngest director of personal training at Flatiron Athletic Club, which was named "Best Gym in America" by *Men's Journal*. Two years later she was honored with the Pursuit of Excellence Award, a grant given to two trainers annually by the National Academy of Sports Medicine. Allison has been featured in *Fitness Business* and *Athletic Business* for her career accomplishments, and she is regularly called upon by local and national publications for her expertise in the field of strength training. She holds a master of science degree in exercise science and multiple certifications through the National Academy of Sports Medicine and USA Triathlon.

Allison's ability to create effective, efficient workouts that improve athletic performance has been featured in *Shape* magazine, *Bicycling*, the *Denver Post*, and Bob Greene's workout DVD *8 Week Total Body Makeover*. Allison's first book, *The Gluten*

Free Fat Loss Plan, was published in May 2011. She has written prolifically on the topic of strength and conditioning and is frequently asked to guest-blog on popular fitness Web sites.

Allison lives in Denver with her husband, Brian, and dog, Muppet. In her spare time she sings with a professional chamber choir and experiments with trying to sit still.

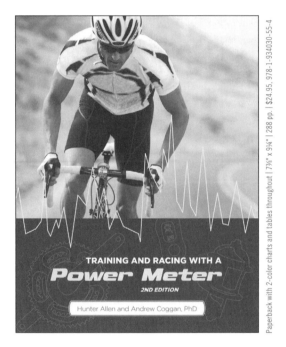
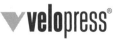